# Low Cholesterol Recipes Book UK 2022

Subtitle: The Ultimate Hearth Healthy Cookbook and Guide on How to Lower Your Cholesterol with Proven, Easy and Delicious Recipes for a Sustainable Healthy Life. 30 Day Meal Plan.

**Author:** Patricia Jones

# Contents

# Introduction

**Causes and Symptoms of Heart Diseases – Everything You Need To Know About Cholesterol and Why Having High Cholesterol Is So Dangerous**

There's a lot of misinformation and misunderstanding about cholesterol and the relationship that it has with people's health. Many people are told that they have high cholesterol, but don't have a proper understanding of what it involves, what causes it, and why it is dangerous to them.

Getting to grips with this is crucial if you are having problems with your cholesterol levels and you need to take control of them. Cholesterol is a waxy substance that is formed in the blood, and it is an important tool that your body uses to build healthy cells – so some cholesterol is absolutely necessary and should be present in your body. It is formed in the liver, and is found in all cells in the body. Some foods also contain cholesterol, especially meat and dairy, and you do require some to survive. However, having a lot of cholesterol in your body is dangerous, and will increase the risk of heart disease.

Essentially, high cholesterol is dangerous because it creates fatty deposits in the blood. As these increase in size, they restrict the blood flowing through your arteries, increasing your blood pressure. If a deposit then breaks away suddenly, it can cause a blood clot, and this may lead to a stroke or a heart attack.

High cholesterol is usually a result of lifestyle choices and poor diet, although it is possible to inherit high cholesterol as well. Whatever the cause, eating well and exercising regularly may help to tackle high cholesterol problems and improve your health.

One of the things that makes high cholesterol particularly dangerous is that it has no symptoms, so you cannot watch out for it yourself. It's possible for you to have high cholesterol for years without realising it. The only way to detect cholesterol issues is through a blood test done by a doctor, and it's useful to have regular screenings throughout a person's life. Even children should be screened on a fairly frequent basis to reduce the risk of heart problems.

Many people will be tested for cholesterol every five years, but if your levels are abnormal or you are over 65, you may be invited to annual tests, as you will be considered "high risk." In some instances, it may be necessary to take medication for high cholesterol problems, but in general, cholesterol is managed via lifestyle choices.

Cholesterol levels are measured in a number of different ways. A test will look at your total cholesterol, your low-density lipoprotein (LDL), your high-density lipoprotein (HDL), your non-HDL (total cholesterol minus HDL), and your Triglycerides, which is a secondary form of fat sometimes found in the blood that increases the risk of heart disease.

In general, LDL cholesterol is considered "bad" and HDL is "good." HDL helps to remove cholesterol from your arteries and reduces your overall risk of heart disease and strokes. It's important not to collate all cholesterol with "bad" or "good," but to understand how it is functioning within your body.

# The Latest Scientific Research on The Low Cholesterol Diet and Weight Loss

**What Is An Ideal Cholesterol Measurement?**

Below are the ideal ranges for the various types of cholesterol:

**In someone 19 or younger:**

Total cholesterol: less than 170 mg/dL (milligrams per decilitre)

Non-HDL: less than 120 mg/dL

LDL: less than 100 mg/dL

HDL: more than 45 mg/dL

**In men over 20 years old:**

Total cholesterol: 125-200 mg/dL (milligrams per decilitre)

Non-HDL: less than 130 mg/dL

LDL: less than 100 mg/dL

HDL: more than 40 mg/dL

**In women over 20 years old:**

Total cholesterol: 125-200 mg/dL (milligrams per decilitre)

Non-HDL: less than 130 mg/dL

LDL: less than 100 mg/dL

HDL: more than 50 mg/dL

In general, doctors count anything over 240 mg/dL as high risk, with anything between 200-239 mg/dL being borderline risk. Be aware of this and understand your own numbers when your doctor gives them to you.

## Does Being Overweight Matter?

High cholesterol levels are often associated with obesity, and it is widely recognised that being a healthy weight can help to decrease the levels of cholesterol within the body and in turn, lower the risk of strokes and heart conditions. Being obese may reduce your body's ability to deal with cholesterol correctly, and it is thought that being a healthy weight will lower the cholesterol levels in most individuals. If you are overweight, you are likely to have higher levels of LDL cholesterol. Your weight will alter how you process fats, including cholesterol and triglycerides. Your body will produce more triglycerides, and is likely to have increased insulin resistance.

It is important to note that your cholesterol levels are not the only thing that your doctor will take an interest in when checking your health. Although there are some basic parameters that they prefer people to fall within, most doctors now recognise that there are many factors at play when determining someone's risk of heart problems, including their age, weight, blood sugar levels, and blood pressure. If you are at risk due to these other factors, you are more likely to need to address your cholesterol levels and reduce them where possible. In the past, many doctors just used fixed numbers to determine what was and was not safe in terms of cholesterol, but recent discoveries have brought more nuance to these calculations. However, there is certainly still a strong link between obesity and raised levels of cholesterol.

## What Should I Be Doing About It?

In general, high cholesterol is treated by modifying both diet and exercise levels to decrease obesity and help the patient reach a moderate weight level. We are going to look at diet throughout this book, but it's important to acknowledge the role that exercise can play too.

It has been proven that physical activity can reduce both the LDL cholesterol and reduce your blood pressure. Doing about 150 minutes of moderate exercise each week is the optimum, but if that's too much, even ten minutes of exercising per day can help to reduce your cholesterol levels and make you healthier. Other steps include reducing or quitting smoking. Smoking is thought to reduce your levels of HDLs, which are needed to protect you from LDLs. Smoking also damages your arteries, making it easier for fatty deposits to get built up there.

In some cases, a doctor will also prescribe medication to try and reduce your cholesterol levels. Statins are the most commonly prescribed option, but your doctor is likely to encourage you to exercise and improve your diet either prior to or in conjunction with taking this kind of medication. There are some other medicines that can also help with cholesterol, but statins are the most commonly prescribed.

# 4 Highly Effective Diet Tips For Easy And Sustainable Weight Loss

Because weight loss is such an important part of reducing your cholesterol levels, it's going to be crucial to look at effective and sustainable weight loss throughout this book. You will find most of the recipes are geared toward helping people lose weight, but it's also important to find ways to form habits that will aid you and ensure that you keep the weight off once you have lost it. So, how can you lose weight quickly, easily, and sustainably?

## Tip One: Eat Regularly

It might sound counter-intuitive, but one of the best ways to help yourself lose weight is to eat regular, controlled portions throughout the day. It is very tempting to skip meals in an attempt to cut down on how much you eat overall, but this actually leaves you at risk of snacking, feeling perpetually hungry, and over-eating at other times to reward yourself for skipping a meal.

Instead, break your day into regular, controlled meals, and minimise snacking. If you eat at regular times every day, you will find that you burn more calories, and that you aren't tempted to overeat during those meals.

It's good to get a little hungry between meals, because this means that your body will start using up fat reserves, rather than just burning off what you have eaten that day. Eating regular meals will help to ensure you aren't snacking for the sake of it, and that you aren't giving your body more fuel than it needs each day.

## Tip Two: Eat Lots Of Fruit And Vegetables

You are probably already aware that making fruits and vegetables key parts of your diet is important, but let's explore just how important. If you are able to build your meals with these as the major components, you will massively cut down on sugar, carbohydrates, and processed foods, as well as salt. You will start building a diet based on vitamins and nutritionally rich foods, and you will feel healthier in many different ways.

It is challenging to stick with this at first, but the more you are able to, the easier it will get. Our bodies learn to crave sugar if we eat sugar, and if you can get past these cravings, you will start to feel better.

Try to make sure that there are at least two fruits or vegetables in every meal you eat, and increase your portions of these, while decreasing your portions of the other meal's components. For example, instead of having two sandwiches with a little salad on the side, have one sandwich with a larger portion of salad. You don't have to give up the carbohydrate-rich foods entirely – just make them a smaller component of your meals, and give fruits and vegetables the spotlight.

## Tip Three: Focus On Fibre

It can be challenging to stick to a diet if you constantly feel hungry, and carbohydrates make us feel full. If you start cutting back on your carbohydrate intake, you're likely to feel hungry more and more often. You may find that meals don't satisfy you, and you want second helpings all the time – which obviously is not ideal from the perspective of cutting down on your food intake.

The answer to this is fibre. The more fibre you eat, the fuller you will feel, and it's a sustained fullness that won't have you wandering back into the kitchen half an hour later to grab some snacks. Build your meals around fibre, and you'll find yourself far more satisfied, and considerably less hungry.

Fibrous foods include brown bread, brown rice, wholemeal pasta, beans, lentils, peas, oats, and fruits and vegetables. Avoid white rice and white bread, as these contain less fibre, and will not leave you feeling full or satisfied. You'll soon want more food, and this doesn't lead to sustained weight loss.

It's really important to ensure that your meals satisfy you. Going hungry all the time is not the way to lose weight sustainably. You might feel like you can handle it for a while, but eventually – as the motivation wears off – you will slide back into snacking and taking bigger portions. You should instead focus on making sure that your meals satisfy you, because this is sustainable and will make your diet commitment last.

## Tip Four: Drink Water

Drinking water throughout the day can stop you from feeling as hungry. Many people mistake thirst for hunger, and eat when instead they need to drink. We get moisture from food, so this satisfies the craving, and leaves us feeling better even though we haven't got what we needed.

Sipping water can also help to reduce a sense of hunger when you're starting out and the diet is hard. Regularly drink a little bit of water every hour or so, and you'll find you stay hydrated and feel less tempted to snack.

# How to Control Your Cholesterol with Ease

There are a few easy steps you can take to get in control of your cholesterol quickly. Your doctor may have further suggestions, but use these to get back on track if you're worried about your levels.

### Tip One: Reduce Saturated Fats

A lot of cholesterol is diet-based, so you need to make sure you are cutting back on your saturated fats if you are going to reduce your cholesterol levels. In general, saturated fats are found in red meat and dairy products (full fat ones particularly). If you eat a lot of cream, cheese, milk, and red meat, try cutting down.

It is okay to include these foods in some instances, but be aware of how often you are eating them, and significantly reduce the frequency and amount that you consume. Try replacing things like butter with olive oil, which is full of "good" fat, and you might lower your cholesterol by as much as 15%.

### Tip Two: Choose Foods Rich In Omega-3 Fatty Acids

Although omega-3 will not affect your LDL levels, it does affect the overall health of your heart. It is thought that these fatty acids can reduce your blood pressure, making it easier for your blood to flow and reducing the risk of a stroke or heart attack.

Fish is a common source of omega-3, but it can also be found in things like walnuts and flax seeds, which are suitable for those following a vegan diet. If you'd rather eat fish, choose oily options like salmon or mackerel. If you are concerned about the health of your heart, omega-3 is a great property to start including in your diet.

### Tip Three: Cut Back On Trans Fats

Another dangerous source of fat is trans fats, and these tend to be found in fried and baked foods. Cakes, pizzas, cookies, fries, chicken wings, and other foods may contain them. There is a reason that these foods are traditionally labelled unhealthy, and you should be looking to avoid them.

Again, you may not need to completely remove all of these things from your diet, but reducing the frequency with which you eat them will improve your heart health.

## Tip Four: Try To Relax

Cholesterol isn't just related to diet; your stress levels also have a major impact on it. If you are feeling stressed, try to find some ways to ensure that you are relaxing each day. You might find that meditation, yoga, or walking help you to feel calmer. In both the long and the short term, this can reduce your cholesterol levels and may improve other aspects of your health too.

## Tip Five: Include More Spices

If you like flavourful food, you're in luck. Many of the commonly used spices, such as black pepper, cinnamon, cumin, coriander, and garlic can reduce your cholesterol levels. Dust your foods with a little spice, grind some pepper into your meals, and try adding more garlic to your dishes to help cut down your cholesterol. It's thought that eating a clove of garlic every day can reduce your cholesterol levels by nearly ten per cent, although this does depend on what else you eat.

## Tip Six: Cut Back On Alcohol

Alcohol is commonly recognised as causing many health issues. It contains a lot of empty calories, it puts pressure on your organs, and it can increase your cholesterol. Ideally, most people should be drinking less than 14 units of alcohol each week, and should avoid drinking on at least several days each week. If you drink a lot, try to implement some alcohol-free days and reduce the overall amount as much as you can to make yourself healthier.

# Heart Protecting Tips for a Healthier and Longer Life

Protecting the health of your heart is crucial, especially among older people – but anyone can have a heart attack, and even very young people suffer from these tragedies at times. If you're concerned about heart health, particularly because family history puts you at risk, you should consider some of these tips for keeping yourself safe.

## Tip One: Exercise

We already discussed how exercising is an important part of managing cholesterol, but it's also an important part of managing your heart health as a whole. Exercise – even moderate exercise – improves many aspects of your physical health, and your heart health is high on the list. Exercise that increases your heart rate massively increases the health of your heart, while sitting still can have a big, negative impact. The more you are able to move around, increase your pulse rate, and get your blood flowing, the healthier your heart and circulatory system will stay. Try to find ways to start moving and keep moving. You can make exercise part of your life in many different ways. Consider walking to work, jogging around the block, or taking up games of tennis or badminton with friends at weekends. Hit the swimming pool or learn to rock climb, or even put a trampoline in your backyard. There are so many ways that you can make yourself healthier by moving around and getting slim, and this will have an impact on many aspects of your health and well-being, not just your heart.

## Tip Two: Meet Your Friends

It might surprise you, but it is thought that loneliness can contribute to heart disease – and no, it isn't because you're broken hearted. Instead, loneliness is thought to cause the arteries to harden, making them less flexible and increasing the risk of a clot. Harder arteries increase your blood pressure, which makes you more vulnerable to heart problems. More study is needed to fully understand this relationship. It's also thought that loneliness is linked with cortisol, the stress hormone, which may interfere with your circulation and increase the amount of work that your heart needs to do. If you're feeling lonely, try reconnecting with old friends, or joining some clubs and forging new social bonds. Although this link is still tenuous and more research is needed, it's certainly true that feeling good mentally can improve your physical health, so it's well worth considering this if you want to live longer and feel better overall.

## Tip Three: Learn How to Meditate

Meditation is not reserved for yoga studios and new-age office environments where everyone needs to be on the same page. Meditation can make a big difference to your life and attitudes, and can revolutionise how you approach the world. It can also massively reduce your risk of heart disease, as several studies have shown. The University of Iowa recently demonstrated that practising meditation for just twenty minutes per day could make a difference to your blood pressure, which in turn reduces your risk of strokes and heart complications.

It can be challenging to make time to meditate in today's busy world, but it's important as well. Try to find ways to fit meditation into your work-life balance. You might decide to meditate after work, before you leave, or during your lunch break. Even if you cannot get meditation into your schedule every single day, doing some is better than doing none! There are many videos that will teach you how to meditate online.

# Tips on Making Absolutely Delicious Low Cholesterol Meals

Let's move on to diet. Diet is probably one of the biggest – if not the biggest – determiner in your cholesterol levels, and taking control of what you eat is going to be crucial. Remember, you want to be decreasing LDLs and increasing HDLs, which will in turn further decrease your LDLs.

Before moving on to the recipes you can use to lower your cholesterol, let's look at a few general cooking tips that you can employ when in the kitchen. You may find that you can use these to adapt some of your "family favourite" recipes to suit your new restrictions, or that they just help to guide your future cooking decisions. However you use them, they should make cooking easier.

### Tip One: Start with the Vegetables

Earlier, we mentioned using vegetables to bulk out your meals, but you may find that it actually helps to start with the vegetables, and expand the meal from there. Instead of thinking "shall I have chicken for tea today?" try thinking "shall I eat broccoli?"

This change in your approach will make vegetables the star of the meal. You can use them to build an entire dish, like stuffed peppers, or add a meat that goes well with that vegetable, but make the vegetable the focal point. This may sound minor, but it alters the overall feeling of the meal, and may help you to eat more vegetables.

### Tip Two: Use Pulses and Beans

If you commonly eat meat and you're trying to cut down, you may find that you don't feel satisfied after a meal. Although this is likely something you will – to an extent – have to just get used to, pulses and beans can help to mitigate the issue. Try adding lentils, kidney beans, or peas to a meal to make yourself feel fuller afterwards. This can go a long way to mitigating your sense of a meal being unsatisfying.

### Tip Three: Swap Your Fats

If you often cook with butter, look at alternative fats that will allow you to make the same meals but without the high cholesterol. Olive oil is often a good alternative, and many buttery meals can be made using olive oil instead.

You can even drizzle olive oil over mashed potatoes instead of using butter, or make gravy with it. Chill it in the fridge and it becomes spreadable, or you can dip bread in warm olive oil as an alternative to butter. Another option is to swap to almond butter, which you'll find recommended in the following recipes. These alternatives all offer great ways to make many of your recipes lower in cholesterol and more suitable for your new diet.

## Tip Four: Bump Up The Spices

We already mentioned how spices can help to reduce your cholesterol, so implement this in your kitchen. This is one of the easiest ways to make your foods better for you, as it takes very little extra work, doesn't restrict your diet, and should make your meals taste better too. Try adding lots of garlic to your meals. Garlic can be eaten raw, or lightly fried to make it fragrant and mild. Almost any meal can include garlic, and it is easy to disguise it with more powerful flavours if you don't particularly enjoy the taste. Bear in mind that raw garlic has a strong taste, but cooked garlic is much subtler.

## Tip Five: Try Probiotics

Some research has indicated that probiotics and good gut health can have an impact on cholesterol levels. It might not seem like your guts and your heart are closely connected, but actually, your gut has a massive impact on what goes into your bloodstream, and in turn, what impacts on your heart. Some probiotics may absorb the cholesterol themselves, preventing it from being passed into the bloodstream, while others convert it into another compound entirely (coprostanol). This will pass through the body without being absorbed. Other probiotics may break down the bile salts in the guts, and cholesterol is required to produce more bile. Cholesterol in the bloodstream will be directed to this purpose, reducing its overall presence in the blood and decreasing the risk of clots. More research is needed to better understand the role that probiotics play in combating high cholesterol, but it's worth talking to your doctor and looking for ways to include things like live yoghurt in your meals. You may be able to use it as a substitute in dishes that require cream or cream cheese, for example. Probiotics may also play a role in weight loss, as they can have an impact on your metabolism. This can improve the overall health of your heart, not just your cholesterol levels. You should speak to your doctor before you add large amounts of probiotics to your meals, however. Although most are safe and beneficial, getting too much of one could cause stomach upset and cramps, so it's best to check with a health practitioner.

# Breakfast Recipes

# Kiwi Smoothie

Servings|2   Time|10 minutes
**Nutritional Content (per serving):**
Cal| 213 Fat| 3.8g Protein| 3.6g Carbs| 46.9g Fibre| 8g Cholesterol| 0mg

## Ingredients:

- Kiwis (4, peeled and sliced)
- Unsweetened almond milk (360 millilitres)
- Small bananas (2, peeled)
- Ice cubes (4-6)

## Directions:

1. Add all the ingredients in a high-power blender and pulse until creamy.
2. Pour the smoothie into two glasses and serve immediately.

# Kale Smoothie

Servings|2   Time|10 minutes
**Nutritional Content (per serving):**
Cal| 158 Fat| 13.4g Protein| 2.8g Carbs| 9.5g Fibre| 4.9g Cholesterol| 0mg

## Ingredients:

- Fresh kale (55 grams, chopped)
- Avocado (½, peeled, pitted, and chopped)
- Celery stalks (1, chopped)
- Chilled unsweetened almond milk (480 millilitres)

## Directions:

1. Add all the ingredients in a high-power blender and pulse until creamy.
2. Pour the smoothie into two glasses and serve immediately.

# Strawberry & Banana Smoothie Bowl

Servings|2   Time|10 minutes
**Nutritional Content (per serving):**
Cal| 155 Fat| 1.7g Protein| 2.4g Carbs| 37.1g Fibre| 5.8g Cholesterol| 0mg

## Ingredients:

- ❖ Fresh strawberries (250 grams, hulled)
- ❖ frozen bananas (2, peeled)
- ❖ Unsweetened almond milk (120 millilitres)

## Directions:

1. In a high-power blender, add strawberries, bananas and almond milk and pulse until smooth.
2. Pour into two serving bowls and serve immediately with your favourite topping.

# Beet & Berries Smoothie Bowl

Servings|1   Time|10 minutes
**Nutritional Content (per serving):**
Cal| 266 Fat| 4.2g Protein| 25.3g Carbs| 31.4g Fibre| 6.9g Cholesterol| 63mg

## Ingredients:

- ❖ Beets (150 grams, peeled and chopped)
- ❖ Unsweetened protein powder (30 grams)
- ❖ Fresh strawberries (125 grams)
- ❖ Fresh cranberries (25 grams)
- ❖ Unsweetened almond milk (120 millilitres)

## Directions:

3. Add all the ingredients in a high-power blender and pulse until smooth.
4. Pour into a serving bowl and serve immediately with your favourite topping.

# Blueberry Chia Pudding

Servings|2   Time|10 minutes
**Nutritional Content (per serving):**
Cal| 148 Fat| 8.6g Protein| 4.8g Carbs| 21g Fibre| 8.2g Cholesterol| 0mg

**Ingredients:**

- ❖ Unsweetened almond milk (120 millilitres)
- ❖ Almond extract (1¼ millilitres)
- ❖ Chia seeds (20 grams)
- ❖ Light maple syrup (10 grams)
- ❖ Fresh blueberries (45 grams)

**Directions:**

1. In a serving bowl, blend together almond milk, chia seed, maple syrup and almond extract.
2. Cover the bowl and refrigerate for at least 8 hours.
3. While serving, stir the mixture well.
4. Stir in blueberries and serve.

# Berries Muesli

Servings|2   Time|10 minutes
**Nutritional Content (per serving):**
Cal| 206 Fat| 5.5g Protein| 5.3g Carbs| 38.8g Fibre| 8.6g Cholesterol| 0mg

**Ingredients:**

- ❖ Muesli (85 grams)
- ❖ Fresh raspberries (125 grams)
- ❖ Unsweetened almond milk (360 millilitres)

**Directions:**

1. Divide muesli into serving bowls and top with raspberries.
2. Pour in almond milk and serve.

# Apple Porridge

Servings|4   Time|15 minutes
**Nutritional Content (per serving):**
Cal| 169 Fat| 8.8g Protein| 3.7g Carbs| 22.4g Fibre| 4.9g Cholesterol| 0mg

## Ingredients:

- ❖ Unsweetened almond milk (480 millilitres)
- ❖ Large apples (2, peeled, cored and grated)
- ❖ Walnuts (20 grams), chopped)
- ❖ Sunflower seeds (30 grams)
- ❖ Vanilla extract (2½ millilitres)
- ❖ Pinch of ground cinnamon

## Directions:

1. In a large-sized saucepan, blend together the milk, walnuts, sunflower seeds, apple, vanilla and cinnamon over medium-low heat and cook for about 3-5 minutes.
2. Serve warm with your favourite topping.

# Seeds Porridge

Servings|2   Time|25 minutes

**Nutritional Content (per serving):**

Cal| 142 Fat| 9.4g Protein| 5g Carbs| 11.6g Fibre| 8.7g Cholesterol| 0mg

## Ingredients:

- Coconut flour (25 grams)
- Flaxseed meal (20 grams)
- Salt, as required
- Unsweetened almond milk (360 millilitres)
- Chia seeds (20 grams)
- Ground cinnamon (5 grams)
- Liquid stevia (10-15 drops)
- Vanilla extract (5 millilitres)

## Directions:

1. In a bowl, blend together coconut flour, chia seeds, flaxseed meal, cinnamon and salt.
2. Add the stevia and almond milk and stir until well blended.
3. Refrigerate, covered overnight before serving.

# Quinoa Porridge

Servings|4  Time|20 minutes
**Nutritional Content (per serving):**
Cal| 362 Fat| 20.1g Protein| 8.4g Carbs| 33.7g Fibre| 3.4g Cholesterol| 0mg

## Ingredients:

- Unsweetened coconut milk (480 millilitres)
- Uncooked quinoa flakes (190 grams, rinsed)
- Water (480 millilitres)
- Almond butter (20 grams)
- Pinch of salt

## Directions:

1. In a saucepan, add coconut milk and water over medium-high heat and bring to a boil.
2. Add the almond butter and stir until well blended.
3. Stir in the quinoa and salt and cook for about 3-5 minutes, stirring continuously.
4. Remove the saucepan of quinoa from heat and set aside, covered for about 2-3 minutes before serving.

# Spiced Quinoa Porridge

Servings|4   Time|25 minutes
**Nutritional Content (per serving):**
Cal| 273 Fat| 12g Protein| 8.1g Carbs| 34.7g Fibre| 5.3g Cholesterol| 0mg

## Ingredients:

- ❖ Uncooked quinoa (190 grams, rinsed)
- ❖ Unsweetened coconut milk (125 millilitres)
- ❖ Ground cinnamon (5 grams)
- ❖ Ground nutmeg (2½ grams)
- ❖ Almonds (10 grams, chopped)
- ❖ Water (480 millilitres)
- ❖ Vanilla extract (2½ millilitres)
- ❖ Lemon peel (2½ grams, grated)
- ❖ Liquid stevia (10-12 drops)
- ❖ Ground ginger (2½ grams)
- ❖ Pinch of ground cloves

## Directions:

1. In a large-sized saucepan, blend together the quinoa, water, and vanilla extract over medium heat and bring to a boil.
2. Now adjust the heat to low and simmer, covered for about 15 minutes or until all the liquid is absorbed, stirring occasionally.
3. In the pan with the quinoa, add the coconut milk, lemon peel, stevia, and spices and stir to combine.
4. Immediately remove from heat and fluff the quinoa with a fork.
5. Serve with a topping of chopped almonds.

# Bulgur Porridge

Servings|4   Time|35 minutes
## Nutritional Content (per serving):

Cal| 363 Fat| 9.3g Protein| 16.9g Carbs| 57g Fibre| 10.4g Cholesterol| 12mg

## Ingredients:

- Low-fat milk (960 millilitres)
- Dried cherries (85 grams)
- Almonds (50 gram, sliced)
- Bulgur (190 grams)
- Dried cherries (85 grams)

## Directions:

1. In a medium-sized saucepan, add milk, bulgur, cherries and salt over medium-high heat and bring to a boil.
2. Now adjust the heat to medium and cook for about 10-15 minutes or until the bulgur is tender, stirring frequently.
3. Serve warm with the topping of almonds.

# Barley Porridge

Servings|3 · Time|1 hour
**Nutritional Content (per serving):**
Cal| 321 Fat| 7g Protein| 9g Carbs| 58.5g Fibre| 12.3g Cholesterol| 0mg

## Ingredients:

- Water (70 millilitres)
- Walnuts (25 grams)
- Ground cinnamon (5 grams)
- Ground nutmeg (1¼ grams)
- Pearl barley (200 grams)
- Light maple syrup (20 grams)
- Unsweetened almond milk (240 millilitres

## Directions:

1. In a saucepan, add the water over high heat and bring to a boil.
2. Add the barley and again bring to a boil.
3. Now adjust the heat to low and simmer, covered for about 35-40 minutes or until most of the liquid is absorbed.
4. Add the walnuts, maple syrup, cinnamon and nutmeg and stir to combine.
5. Stir in 120 millilitres of almond milk and cook for about 2-3 minutes.
6. Stir in the remaining almond milk and remove from heat.
7. Serve warm.

# Buckwheat Porridge

Servings|2   Time|17 minutes
**Nutritional Content (per serving):**
Cal| 269 Fat| 2.5g Protein| 8.1g Carbs| 59.1g Fibre| 9.5g Cholesterol| 0mg

## Ingredients:

- Buckwheat groats (120 grams)
- Water (240 millilitres)
- Unsweetened almond milk (60 millilitres)
- 1Apple (1, cored and grated)
- Ground cinnamon (2½ grams)
- Vanilla extract (1¼ millilitres)

## Directions:

1. In a large-sized bowl, soak buckwheat groats in 240 millilitres of water overnight.
2. Drain the buckwheat and rinse well.
3. In a non-stick saucepan, add the buckwheat, apple, water and almond milk over medium-low heat and cook for about 10-12 minutes, stirring frequently.
4. Remove the saucepan of porridge from heat and stir in the cinnamon and vanilla extract.
5. Serve hot with your favourite fruit topping.

# Oatmeal Yoghurt Bowl

Servings|2  Time|10 minutes
**Nutritional Content (per serving):**
Cal| 232 Fat| 3.9g Protein| 9.7g Carbs| 41.5g Fibre| 5.6g Cholesterol| 1mg

## Ingredients:

- ❖ Gluten-free old-fashioned oats (100 grams)
- ❖ Fat-free plain Greek yoghurt (150 grams)
- ❖ Water (480 millilitres)
- ❖ Ground cinnamon (1¼ grams)
- ❖ Fresh strawberries (65 grams, hulled and sliced)

## Directions:

1. In a saucepan, add water over medium heat and bring to a boil.
2. Stir in the oats and cook for about 5 minutes, stirring occasionally.
3. Remove the pan of oats from heat and stir in half of the fat-free yoghurt and cinnamon.
4. Serve with the topping of strawberry slices.

# Blueberry Oatmeal

Servings|2   Time|20 minutes
## Nutritional Content (per serving):
Cal| 304 Fat| 3.8g Protein| 7g Carbs| 57.8g Fibre| 2.3g Cholesterol| 0mg

## Ingredients:

- Unsweetened almond milk (480 millilitres)
- Light maple syrup (35 grams)
- Gluten-free oats (100 grams)
- Frozen blueberries (100 grams)
- Fresh lemon juice (15 millilitres)

## Directions:

1. In a saucepan, add the almond milk, oats and blueberries over medium heat and cook for about 8-10 minutes, stirring occasionally.
2. Remove the saucepan of oatmeal from heat and stir in the maple syrup and lemon juice.
3. Serve warm.

# Baked Oatmeal

Servings|6 · Time|1 hour
**Nutritional Content (per serving):**
Cal| 324 Fat| 18.3g Protein| 7.6g Carbs| 34.9g Fibre| 5.6g Cholesterol| 0mg

## Ingredients:

- ❖ Flaxseed meal (10 grams)
- ❖ Unsweetened almond milk (720 millilitres)
- ❖ Coconut oil (25 grams, melted and cooled)
- ❖ Salt (1¼ grams)
- ❖ Mixed nuts (100 grams, chopped)
- ❖ Water (45 millilitres)
- ❖ Light maple syrup (70 grams)
- ❖ Vanilla extract (10 millilitres)
- ❖ Ground cinnamon (5 grams)
- ❖ Baking powder (4 grams)
- ❖ Gluten-free old-fashioned rolled oats (200 grams)

## Directions:

1. In a large-sized bowl, add the flaxseed meal and water and beat until well blended. Set aside for about 5 minutes.
2. In the bowl of flax mixture, add the remaining ingredients except for the oats and nuts and mix until well blended.
3. Add the oats and nuts and gently stir to combine.
4. Place the mixture into a lightly greased 8x8-inch baking dish and spread in an even layer.
5. Cover the baking dish with plastic wrap and refrigerate for about 8 hours.
6. Preheat your oven to 180 °C. Arrange a rack in the middle of the oven.
7. Remove the baking dish from refrigerator and set aside at room temperature for 15-20 minutes.
8. Remove the plastic wrap and stir the oatmeal mixture well.
9. Bake for approximately 45 minutes.
10. Serve warm.

# Tofu & Veggie Scramble

Servings|2   Time|30 minutes
**Nutritional Content (per serving):**
Cal| 225 Fat| 13.1g Protein| 17.5g Carbs| 15g Fibre| 4.5g Cholesterol| 0mg

## Ingredients:

- ❖ Olive oil (10 millilitres)
- ❖ Small Pepper (1, seeded and finely chopped)
- ❖ Firm tofu (380 grams, pressed, drained and crumbled)
- ❖ Salt, as required
- ❖ Small onion (1, finely chopped)
- ❖ Tomatoes ((200 grams, finely chopped)
- ❖ Pinch of cayenne pepper
- ❖ Pinch of ground turmeric

## Directions:

1. In a non-stick wok, heat oil over medium heat and sauté the onion and pepper for about 4-5 minutes.
2. Add the tomatoes and cook for about 1-2 minutes.
3. Add the tofu, turmeric, cayenne pepper and salt and cook for about 6-8 minutes.
4. Serve hot.

# Vanilla Pancakes

Servings|5   Time|30 minutes
**Nutritional Content (per serving):**
Cal| 282 Fat| 17g Protein| 5.1g Carbs| 30.6g Fibre| 4.8g Cholesterol| 0mg

## Ingredients:

- Unsweetened coconut milk (250 millilitres)
- Buckwheat flour (125 grams)
- Baking powder (14 grams)
- Light maple syrup (70 grams)
- Olive oil (15 millilitres)
- Apple cider vinegar (10 millilitres)
- Ground flaxseed (20 grams)
- Salt (1¼ grams)
- Vanilla extract (5 millilitres)

## Directions:

1. In a medium-sized bowl, blend together the coconut milk and vinegar. Set aside.
2. In a large-sized bowl, blend together the flour, flaxseed, baking powder, and salt.
3. Add the coconut milk mixture, maple syrup, and vanilla extract and beat until well blended.
4. In a large-sized non-stick wok, heat oil over medium heat.
5. Place desired amount of the mixture and spread in an even circle.
6. Cook for about 1-2 minutes.
7. Flip and cook for an additional 1 minute.
8. Repeat with the remaining mixture.
9. Serve warm.

# Banana Pancakes

Servings|2   Time|23 minutes
**Nutritional Content (per serving):**
Cal| 181 Fat| 9.6g Protein| 6.8g Carbs| 19g Fibre| 2.9g Cholesterol| 0mg

## Ingredients:

- Gluten-free rolled oats (25 grams)
- Baking soda (1 gram)
- Unsweetened almond milk (120 millilitres)
- Banana (½, peeled and mashed)
- Arrowroot flour (30 grams)
- Baking powder (2 grams)
- Ground cinnamon (1 gram)
- Egg whites (2)
- Almond butter (10 grams)
- Vanilla extract (2½ millilitres)
- Olive oil (15 millilitres)

## Directions:

1. In a large-sized bowl, add the flour, oats, baking soda, baking powder and cinnamon and mix well.
2. In another large-sized bowl, add the almond milk, egg whites, almond butter, mashed banana and vanilla and beat until well blended.
3. Add the flour mixture and mix until well blended.
4. In a large-sized non-stick wok, heat oil over medium heat.
5. Add half of the mixture and cook for about 1-2 minutes per side.
6. Repeat with the remaining mixture.
7. Serve warm.

# Blueberry Waffles

Servings|6   Time|34 minutes
**Nutritional Content (per serving):**
Cal| 403 Fat| 20.6g Protein| 4.8g Carbs| 43.7g Fibre| 8.2g Cholesterol| 0mg

## Ingredients:

- Almond flour (200 grams)
- Cornstarch (15 grams)
- Ground cinnamon (5 grams)
- Light maple syrup (70 grams)
- Unsweetened almond milk (720 millilitres)
- Oat flour (180 grams)
- Baking powder (25 grams)
- Salt (2½ grams)
- Vanilla extract (5 millilitres)
- Fresh blueberries (190 grams)

## Directions:

1. In a large-sized bowl, blend together the flours, cornstarch, baking powder, cinnamon and salt.
2. Add the almond milk and vanilla and mix until just combined.
3. Gently fold in the blueberries.
4. Preheat your waffle iron and then grease it.
5. Place the desired amount of the mixture into the preheated waffle iron and cook for about 5-6 minutes or until golden brown.
6. Repeat with the remaining mixture.
7. Serve warm with the drizzling of extra maple syrup.

# Blueberry Muffins

Servings|5   Time|27 minutes
**Nutritional Content (per serving):**
Cal| 124 Fat| 6.5g Protein| 3.9g Carbs| 11.8g Fibre| 3.4g Cholesterol| 33mg

## Ingredients:

- Gluten-free rolled oats (50 grams)
- Baking soda (2 grams)
- Almond butter (60 grams)
- Egg (1)
- Fresh blueberries (50 grams)

- Almond flour (25 grams)
- Flaxseeds (20 grams)
- Ground cinnamon (2½ grams)
- Banana (20 grams, peeled and mashed)

## Directions:

1. Preheat your oven to 190 ºC. Lightly grease 10 cups of a muffin tin.
2. In a clean blender, place all the ingredients except for the blueberries and pulse until smooth and creamy.
3. Transfer the mixture into a bowl and fold in blueberries.
4. Place the mixture into prepared muffin cups evenly.
5. Bake for approximately 10-12 minutes or until a wooden skewer inserted in the centre comes out clean.
6. Remove the muffin tin from oven and place onto a wire rack to cool for about 9-10 minutes.
7. Carefully invert the muffins onto the wire rack to cool completely before serving.

# Kale Muffins

Servings|6   Time|55 minutes
**Nutritional Content (per serving):**
Cal| 253 Fat| 22.8g Protein| 6.5g Carbs| 7.8g Fibre| 1g Cholesterol| 130mg

## Ingredients:

- ❖ Eggs (6)
- ❖ Arrowroot starch (30 grams)
- ❖ Baking powder (1 gram)
- ❖ Coconut oil (95 grams, melted and cooled slightly)
- ❖ Fresh kale (85 grams, tough ribs removed and sliced thinly)
- ❖ Fresh chives (10 grams, sliced)
- ❖ Coconut flour (45 grams)
- ❖ Baking soda (2 grams)
- ❖ Salt and ground black pepper, as required
- ❖ Unsweetened coconut milk (60-65 millilitres)
- ❖ Medium shallot (1, finely chopped)

## Directions:

1. Preheat your oven to 180 °C. Line a 12 cups standard-sized muffin tin with paper liners.
2. In a clean blender, add eggs and pulse on low speed until whipped.
3. Add the coconut flour, arrowroot starch, baking soda, baking powder, salt, black pepper, coconut oil and coconut milk and pulse until well blended.
4. Transfer the mixture into a large-sized bowl.
5. Add the kale, shallot and chives and stir to combine.
6. Place the mixture into prepared muffin cups evenly.
7. Bake for approximately 35-40 minutes or until tops become golden brown.
8. Remove the muffin tin from oven and place onto a wire rack to cool for about 9-10 minutes.
9. Carefully invert the muffins onto a platter and serve warm.

# Quinoa Bread

Servings|12   Time|1 hour 40 minutes
**Nutritional Content (per serving):**
Cal| 156 Fat| 7.5g Protein| 4.6g Carbs| 19.3g Fibre| 3.1g Cholesterol| 0mg

## Ingredients:

- ❖ Uncooked quinoa (335 grams)
- ❖ Bicarbonate soda (2 grams)
- ❖ Olive oil (60 millilitres)
- ❖ Water (120 millilitres)

- ❖ Uncooked quinoa (335 grams)
- ❖ Salt (1½ grams)
- ❖ Fresh lemon juice (15 millilitres)

## Directions:

1. Soak quinoa in water overnight.
2. Soak the chia seeds in 240 millilitres of water overnight.
3. Then drain the quinoa completely.
4. Preheat oven to 160 °C. Line a loaf pan with parchment paper.
5. In a clean food processor, add soaked chia seeds, drained quinoa and remaining ingredients and pulse for about 3 minutes.
6. Place the mixture into the prepared loaf pan evenly.
7. Bake for approximately 1½ hours or until a wooden skewer inserted in the centre comes out clean.
8. Remove the loaf pan from oven and place onto a wire rack to cool for at least 10-15 minutes.
9. Then invert the bread onto the rack to cool completely before slicing.
10. Cut the bread loaf into desired-sized slices and serve.

# Courgette Bread

Servings|6 · Time|1 hour
**Nutritional Content (per serving):**
Cal| 98 Fat| 5.2g Protein| 1g Carbs| 10.6g Fibre| 2.4g Cholesterol| 0mg

## Ingredients:

- Almond flour (50 grams, sifted)
- Ground cinnamon (2½ grams)
- Banana (200 grams, peeled and mashed)
- Courgette (115 grams, shredded)
- Baking soda (6 grams)
- Ground cardamom (1¼ grams)
- Almond butter (60 grams, softened)
- Vanilla extract (10 millilitres)

## Directions:

1. Preheat oven to 180 °C. Grease a 6x3-inch loaf pan.
2. In a large-sized bowl, blend together the flour, baking soda and spices.
3. In another bowl, add the remaining ingredients except courgette and beat until well blended.
4. Fold in the grated courgette.
5. Transfer the batter into the prepared loaf pan.
6. Bake for approximately 40-45 minutes or until a wooden skewer inserted in the centre comes out clean.
7. Remove from oven and place the loaf pan onto a wire rack to cool for at least 10 minutes.
8. Then invert the bread onto the rack to cool completely before slicing.
9. Cut the bread loaf into desired-sized slices and serve.

# Banana Sandwich

Servings|2 · Time|13 minutes
**Nutritional Content (per serving):**
Cal| 445 Fat| 27.1g Protein| 12.6g Carbs| 48.9g Fibre| 7.8g Cholesterol| 0mg

## Ingredients:

- ❖ Whole-wheat bread slices (2)
- ❖ Banana (1, peeled and sliced)
- ❖ Olive oil (15 millilitres)
- ❖ Peanut butter (30 grams)
- ❖ Ground cinnamon (1½ grams)

## Directions:

1. Arrange the bread slices onto a plate.
2. Spread peanut butter on one side of each bread slice.
3. Place banana slices over one bread slice and sprinkle with cinnamon.
4. Cover with remaining bread slice, peanut butter side down.
5. In a frying pan, heat the oil over medium heat and cook the sandwich for about 1½ minutes per side or until golden brown.
6. Transfer the sandwich onto a plate.
7. Cut into half diagonally and serve.

# Avocado & Chickpeas Toast

Servings|2   Time|17 minutes
**Nutritional Content (per serving):**
Cal| 434 Fat| 29.2g Protein| 9.6g Carbs| 40.3g Fibre| 12.8g Cholesterol| 0mg

## Ingredients:

- ❖ Olive oil (15 millilitres, divided)
- ❖ Ground turmeric (5 grams)
- ❖ Salt and ground black pepper, as required
- ❖ Whole-wheat bread slices (2, toasted)
- ❖ Cooked chickpeas (165 grams)
- ❖ Fresh lemon juice (5 millilitres)
- ❖ Small avocado (1, peeled, pitted and chopped roughly)

## Directions:

1. In a non-stick wok, heat 15 millilitres of oil over medium heat and cook the chickpeas for about 3-4 minutes, stirring continuously.
2. Stir in the turmeric and cook for about 2-3 minutes or until chickpeas are toasted.
3. Remove the wok of chickpeas from heat and stir in the lemon juice, salt and black pepper. Set aside.
4. In a bowl, add the chopped avocado with a pinch of salt and black pepper and with a fork, mash well.
5. Arrange 1 bread slice onto each serving plate.
6. Spread mashed avocado on one side of each bread slice and top with chickpeas.
7. Serve immediately.

# Lunch Recipes

# Apple & Strawberry Salad

Servings|4   Time|15 minutes
**Nutritional Content (per serving):**
Cal| 237 Fat| 16.9g Protein| 1.7g Carbs| 23.1g Fibre| 4.5g Cholesterol| omg

## Ingredients:

### For Salad:

- ❖ Mixed lettuce (150 grams, torn)
- ❖ Fresh strawberries (125 grams, hulled and sliced)
- ❖  Apples (2, cored and sliced)
- ❖ Pecans (30 grams, chopped)

### For Dressing:

- ❖ Balsamic vinegar (45 millilitres)
- ❖ Olive oil (45 millilitres)
- ❖ Light maple syrup (20 grams)
- ❖ Poppy seeds (5 grams)
- ❖ Salt, as required

## Directions:

1. For salad: place all the ingredients in a large-sized salad bowl and mix well.
2. For the dressing, place all the ingredients in a bowl and beat until well blended.
3. Pour the dressing over the salad and toss it all to coat well.
4. Serve immediately.

# Orange & Kale Salad

Servings|2   Time|10 minutes
**Nutritional Content (per serving):**
Cal| 267 Fat| 14.5g Protein| 4.4g Carbs| 34.2g Fibre| 6g Cholesterol| 0mg

## Ingredients:

### For Salad:

- ❖ Fresh kale (170 grams, tough ribs removed and torn)
- ❖ Oranges (2, peeled and segmented)
- ❖ Fresh cranberries (15 grams)

### For Dressing:

- ❖ Olive oil (30 millilitres)
- ❖ Fresh orange juice (30 millilitres)
- ❖ Light maple syrup (5 grams)
- ❖ Salt, as required

## Directions:

1. For salad: place all ingredients in a salad bowl and mix.
2. For dressing: place all ingredients in n another bowl and beat until well blended.
3. Pour the dressing over salad and toss to coat well.
4. Serve immediately.

# Tomato & Greens Salad

Servings|4   Time|10 minutes
**Nutritional Content (per serving):**
Cal| 96 Fat| 7.3g Protein| 2g Carbs| 7.3g Fibre| 2.3g Cholesterol| 0mg

**Ingredients:**

- ❖ Fresh baby greens (180 grams)
- ❖ Cherry tomatoes (350 grams, halved)
- ❖ Fresh orange juice (30 millilitres)
- ❖ Green onions (2, chopped)
- ❖ Extra-virgin olive oil (30 millilitres)
- ❖ Fresh lemon juice (15 millilitres)

**Directions:**

1. Place all the ingredients in a large-sized salad bowl and toss to coat well.
2. Serve immediately.

# Cucumber & Tomato Salad

Servings|4   Time|10 minutes
**Nutritional Content (per serving):**
Cal| 97 Fat| 7.5g Protein| 1.9g Carbs| 7.8g Fibre| 2g Cholesterol| 0mg

**Ingredients:**

- ❖ Tomatoes (400 grams, chopped)
- ❖ Mixed lettuce (80 grams, torn)
- ❖ Olive oil (30 millilitres)
- ❖ Cucumbers (300 grams, chopped)
- ❖ Fresh baby spinach (60 grams)
- ❖ Salt, as required

**Directions:**

1. Place all the ingredients in a large-sized salad bowl and toss to combine.
2. Serve immediately.

# Tomato Soup

Servings|4   Time|30 minutes
**Nutritional Content (per serving):**
Cal| 127 Fat| 4.4g Protein| 4.8g Carbs| 21.5g Fibre| 4.7g Cholesterol| 0mg

## Ingredients:

- Olive oil (15 millilitres)
- Garlic cloves (3, minced)
- Fresh basil ((20 grams, chopped)
- Cayenne powder (1¼ grams)
- Medium onion (1, chopped)
- Tomatoes (1400 grams, chopped)
- Salt, as required

## Directions:

1. In a large-sized soup pan, heat oil over medium heat and sauté the onion and garlic for about 5-6 minutes.
2. Add the tomatoes and cook for about 6-8 minutes, crushing with the back of a spoon occasionally.
3. Stir in the basil, salt and cayenne powder and remove from heat.
4. With a hand blender, puree the soup mixture until smooth.
5. Serve immediately.

# Asparagus Soup

Servings|4   Time|50 minutes
**Nutritional Content (per serving):**
Cal| 86 Fat| 3.8g Protein| 6.1g Carbs| 8.7g Fibre| 3.9g Cholesterol| 0mg

## Ingredients:

- ❖ Olive oil (15 millilitres)
- ❖ Fresh asparagus (690 grams, trimmed and chopped)
- ❖ Salt and ground black pepper, as required
- ❖ Green onions (3, chopped)
- ❖ Low-sodium vegetable broth (960 millilitres)
- ❖ Fresh lemon juice (30 millilitres)

## Directions:

1. In a large-sized saucepan, heat the oil over medium heat and sauté the green onion for 4-5 minutes.
2. Stir in the asparagus and broth and bring to a boil.
3. Now adjust the heat to low and simmer, covered for 25-30 minutes.
4. Remove from heat and set aside to cool slightly.
5. Now, transfer the soup into a high-speed blender in 2 batches and pulse until smooth.
6. Return the soup into the same pan over medium heat and simmer for 4-5 minutes.
7. Stir in the lemon juice, salt, and black pepper and remove from heat.
8. Serve hot.

# Broccoli Soup

Servings|4 · Time|1 hour
**Nutritional Content (per serving):**
Cal| 235 Fat| 17.6g Protein| 5g Carbs| 17.6g Fibre| 7.6g Cholesterol| 0mg

## Ingredients:

- Olive oil (30 millilitres)
- Garlic clove (1, minced)
- Ground cumin (1¼ grams)
- Low-sodium vegetable broth (960 millilitres)
- Avocado (1, peeled, pitted and chopped)
- Onion (60 grams, chopped)
- Fresh thyme (5 grams, chopped)
- Red pepper flakes (1¼ grams)
- Medium heads broccoli (2, cut into florets)

## Directions:

1. In a large-sized soup pan, heat oil over medium heat and sauté the onion for about 4-5 minutes.
2. Add the garlic, thyme and spices and sauté for about 1 minute more.
3. Add the broccoli and cook for about 3-4 minutes.
4. Stir in the broth and bring to a boil over high heat.
5. Now adjust the heat to medium-low.
6. Cover the soup pan and cook for about 32-35 minutes.
7. Remove from heat and set aside to cool slightly.
8. In a blender, place the mixture in batches with avocado and pulse until smooth.
9. Serve immediately.

# Cauliflower Soup

Servings|4   Time|35 minutes
**Nutritional Content (per serving):**
Cal| 227 Fat| 16.4g Protein| 5.3g Carbs| 14.2g Fibre| 3.8g Cholesterol| 0mg

## Ingredients:

- Olive oil (30 millilitres)
- Carrots (2, peeled and chopped)
- Garlic cloves (2, minced)
- Ground turmeric (5 grams)
- Ground cumin (5 grams)
- Cauliflower head (1, chopped)
- Unsweetened coconut milk (250 millilitres)
- Fresh chives ((10 grams, chopped)
- Onion (1, chopped)
- Celery stalks (2, chopped)
- Serrano pepper (1, chopped)
- Ground coriander (5 grams)
- Red pepper flakes (1¼ grams)
- Low-sodium vegetable broth (960 millilitres)
- Salt and ground black pepper, as required

## Directions:

1. In a large-sized saucepan, heat the oil over medium heat and sauté the onion, carrot, and celery for 5-6 minutes.
2. Add the garlic, Serrano pepper and spices and sauté for about 1 minute.
3. Add the cauliflower and cook for 5 minutes, stirring occasionally.
4. Add the broth and coconut milk and bring to a boil over medium-high heat.
5. Now adjust the heat to low and simmer for 15 minutes.
6. Season the soup with salt and black pepper and serve hot with a topping of chives.

# Chicken Lettuce Wraps

Servings|5   Time|15 minutes
**Nutritional Content (per serving):**
Cal| 238 Fat| 8.5g Protein| 33.5g Carbs| 4.9g Fibre| 1.2g Cholesterol| 90mg

## Ingredients:

- ❖ Cooked ground chicken (570 grams)
- ❖ Fresh parsley (10 grams, chopped)
- ❖ Romaine lettuce leaves (10)
- ❖ Carrots (225 grams, peeled and julienned)
- ❖ Fresh lime juice (30 millilitres)

## Directions:

1. Arrange the lettuce leaves onto serving plates.
2. Place the cooked chicken and carrot over each lettuce leaf.
3. Drizzle with lime juice and serve immediately.

# Salmon Lettuce Wraps

Servings|4   Time|20 minutes
**Nutritional Content (per serving):**
Cal| 152 Fat| 6.3g Protein| 20.1g Carbs| 4.6g Fibre| 0.8g Cholesterol| 44mg

## Ingredients:

- ❖ Large lettuce leaves (8)
- ❖ Carrot (1, peeled and julienned)
- ❖ Cucumber (1, julienned)
- ❖ Cooked salmon (400 grams, chopped)
- ❖ Fresh chives (5 grams, minced)

## Directions:

1. Arrange lettuce leaves onto serving plates.
2. Divide the salmon pieces, carrot and cucumber over the leaves evenly.
3. Garnish with chives and serve immediately.

# Turkey Burgers

Servings|6   Time|25 minutes
**Nutritional Content (per serving):**
Cal| 147 Fat| 8.1g Protein| 15.5g Carbs| 5.2g Fibre| 0.9g Cholesterol| 54mg

## Ingredients:

- Fresh ginger (1 (5-centimetres) piece, grated)
- Medium onion (1, grated)
- Fresh mint leaves (10 grams, finely chopped)
- Salt and ground black pepper, as required
- Lean ground turkey (455 grams)
- Garlic cloves (2, minced)
- Ground coriander (5 grams)
- Ground cumin (5 grams)
- Olive oil (15 millilitres)
- Fresh spinach (200 grams)

## Directions:

1. Preheat the broiler of your oven. Lightly grease a broiler pan.
2. In a large-sized bowl, squeeze the juice of ginger.
3. Add remaining ingredients and mix until well blended.
4. Make equal-sized burgers from the mixture.
5. Arrange the patties onto the prepared broiler pan and broil for about 5 minutes per side.
6. Serve the burgers alongside the spinach.

# Beef Burgers

Servings|4   Time|27 minutes
## Nutritional Content (per serving):
Cal| 271Fat| 17.2g Protein| 26.5g Carbs| 4.1g Fibre| 1.5g Cholesterol| 98mg

## Ingredients:

- Lean ground beef (455 grams)
- Small onion (½, chopped)
- Sun-dried tomatoes (15 grams, chopped)
- Salt and ground black pepper, as required
- Fresh baby kale (180 grams)
- Fresh spinach (30 grams, chopped)
- Egg (1, beaten)
- Low-fat feta cheese (30 grams, crumbled)
- Olive oil (30 millilitres)

## Directions:

1. In a large-sized bowl, add all the ingredients except for oil and kale and mix until well blended.
2. Make 4 equal-sized patties from the mixture.
3. In a cast-iron wok, heat oil over medium-high heat and cook the patties for about 5-6 minutes per side or until desired doneness.
4. Serve alongside the kale.

# Tofu & Oats Burgers

Servings|4   Time|31 minutes
**Nutritional Content (per serving):**
Cal| 298 Fat| 16.6g Protein| 16.1g Carbs| 25g Fibre| 8g Cholesterol| 0mg

## Ingredients:

- ❖ Firm tofu (455 grams, drained, pressed and crumbled)
- ❖ Flaxseeds (35 grams)
- ❖ Medium onion (1, finely chopped)
- ❖ Ground cumin (5 grams)
- ❖ Salt and ground black pepper, as required
- ❖ Gluten-free rolled oats (75 grams)
- ❖ Frozen spinach (60 grams, thawed)
- ❖ Garlic cloves (4, minced)
- ❖ Red pepper flakes (5 grams)
- ❖ Olive oil (30 millilitres)
- ❖ Fresh salad greens (200 grams)

## Directions:

1. In a large-sized bowl, add all the ingredients except oil and salad greens and mix until well blended.
2. Set aside for about 10 minutes.
3. Make desired size patties from the mixture.
4. In a non-stick frying pan, heat the oil over medium heat and cook the patties for 6-8 minutes per side.
5. Serve these patties alongside the salad greens.

# Tuna Stuffed Avocado

Servings|2   Time|15 minutes
**Nutritional Content (per serving):**
Cal| 380 Fat| 27.8g Protein| 20.2g Carbs| 14.8g Fibre| 6.9g Cholesterol| 27mg

## Ingredients:

- Large avocado (1, halved and pitted)
- Fat-free mayonnaise (45 grams)
- Onion (10 grams, finely chopped)
- Water-packed tuna (1 (140-gram) can, drained and flaked)
- Fresh lime juice (30 millilitres)
- Salt and ground black pepper, as required

## Directions:

1. Carefully, remove about some flesh from each avocado half.
2. Arrange the avocado halves onto a platter and drizzle each with 5 millilitres of lime juice.
3. Chop the avocado flesh and transfer into a bowl.
4. In the bowl of avocado flesh, add tuna, mayonnaise, onion, remaining lemon juice, salt, and black pepper and stir to combine.
5. Divide the tuna mixture in both avocado halves evenly and serve immediately.

# Chickpeas Stuffed Avocado

Servings|2  Time|15 minutes
**Nutritional Content (per serving):**
Cal| 411 Fat| 30.7g Protein| 9.4g Carbs| 29g Fibre| 11.5g Cholesterol| 0mg

## Ingredients:

- Large avocado (1, halved and pitted)
- Celery stalk (1, chopped)
- Garlic clove (1, minced)
- Fresh lemon juice (15 millilitres)
- Fresh coriander (5 grams, chopped)
- Cooked chickpeas (150 grams)
- Walnuts ((25 grams, chopped)
- Green onion (1, sliced)
- Olive oil (5 millilitres)
- Salt and ground black pepper, as required

## Directions:

1. With a spoon, scoop out the flesh from each avocado half.
2. Then, cut half of the avocado flesh in equal-sized cubes.
3. In a large-sized bowl, add avocado cubes and remaining ingredients except for sunflower seeds and cilantro and toss to coat well.
4. Stuff each avocado half with chickpeas mixture evenly.
5. Serve immediately with the garnishing of coriander.

# Veggie Kebabs

Servings|4  Time|30 minutes
**Nutritional Content (per serving):**
Cal| 123 Fat| 7.9g Protein| 4.1g Carbs| 12.8g Fibre| 3.7g Cholesterol| 0mg

## Ingredients:

- Garlic cloves (2, minced)
- Cayenne pepper (1½ grams)
- Fresh lemon juice (30 millilitres)
- Large Courgettes (2, cut into thick slices)
- Peppers (2, seeded and cubed)
- Fresh basil (10 grams, minced)
- Salt and ground black pepper, as required
- Olive oil (30 millilitres)
- Large button mushrooms (8, quartered)

## Directions:

1. For marinade: in a large-sized bowl, add garlic, basil, cayenne, salt, black pepper, oil and lemon juice and mix until well blended.
2. Add the vegetables and toss to coat well.
3. Cover the bowl of vegetables and refrigerate to marinate for at least 6-8 hours.
4. Preheat your grill to medium-high heat. Generously grease the grill grate.
5. Remove the vegetables from the bowl and thread onto pre-soaked wooden skewers.
6. Place the skewers onto the grill and cook for about 8-10 minutes, flipping occasionally.
7. Serve hot.

# Vegetarian Taco Bowl

Servings|2   Time|10 minutes
**Nutritional Content (per serving):**
Cal| 236   Fat| 1.5g Protein| 12.5g Carbs| 47g Fibre| 13.2g Cholesterol| 0mg

## Ingredients:

- Pepper (1, seeded and chopped)
- Cooked red kidney beans (130 grams)
- Lettuce (100 grams, chopped)
- Fresh lime juice (15 millilitres)
- Onion (1, sliced)
- Cooked black beans (130 grams)
- Frozen corn (65 grams, thawed)
- Jalapeño pepper (1, seeded and minced)

## Directions:

1. Divide the beans, corn, veggies, lettuce and jalapeño pepper into serving bowls.
2. Drizzle with lime juice and serve.

# Nutty Brussels Sprout

Servings|2   Time|30 minutes
**Nutritional Content (per serving):**
Cal| 170 Fat| 12.9g Protein| 5.3g Carbs| 13.1g Fibre| 4.9g Cholesterol| 0mg

## Ingredients:

- Brussels sprouts (225 grams, halved)
- Red pepper flakes (2½ grams)
- Fresh lime juice (15 millilitres)
- Pine nuts (15 grams)

- Olive oil (15 millilitres)
- Garlic cloves (2, minced)
- Salt and ground black pepper, as required

## Directions:

1. In a large-sized saucepan of boiling water, arrange a steamer basket.
2. Place asparagus in steamer basket and steam, covered for about 6-8 minutes.
3. Drain the asparagus well.
4. In a large-sized wok, heat the oil over medium heat and sauté the garlic and red pepper flakes for about 40 seconds.
5. Stir in the Brussels sprouts, salt and black pepper and sauté for about 4-5 minutes.
6. Stir in lime juice and sauté for about 1 minute more.
7. Stir in the pine nuts and serve hot.

# Broccoli with Peppers

Servings|4   Time|25 minutes
**Nutritional Content (per serving):**
Cal| 125 Fat| 7.5g Protein| 2.9g Carbs| 14.3g Fibre| 3.2g Cholesterol| 0mg

## Ingredients:

- Olive oil (30 millilitres)
- Peppers (3, seeded and sliced)
- Salt and ground black pepper, as required
- Garlic cloves (4, minced)
- Large onion (1, sliced)
- broccoli florets (180 grams)
- Low-sodium vegetable broth (60 millilitres)

## Directions:

1. In a large-sized wok, heat the oil over medium heat and sauté the garlic for about 1 minute.
2. Add the onion, broccoli and peppers and stir fry for about 5 minutes.
3. Add the broth and stir fry for about 4 minutes more.
4. Serve hot.

# Aubergine Curry

**Nutritional Content (per serving):**
Cal| 245 Fat| 17.2g Protein| 4g Carbs| 19.4g Fibre| 7.8g Cholesterol| 0mg

## Ingredients:

- Olive oil (15 millilitres)
- Garlic cloves (2, minced)
- Serrano pepper (1, seeded and minced)
- Cayenne pepper (1¼ grams)
- Medium tomato (1, finely chopped)
- Unsweetened coconut milk (250 millilitres)
- Medium onion (1, finely chopped)
- Fresh ginger (5 grams, minced)
- Curry powder (5 grams)
- Salt, as required
- Large aubergine (1, cubed)
- Fresh coriander (10 grams, chopped)

## Directions:

1. In a large-sized wok, heat oil over medium heat and sauté the onion for 8-9 minutes.
2. Add the garlic, garlic, Serrano pepper, curry powder, cayenne pepper, and salt and sauté for 1 minute.
3. Add the tomato and cook for 3-4 minutes, crushing with the back of the spoon.
4. Add the aubergine and salt and cook for 1 minute, stirring occasionally.
5. Stir in the coconut milk and bring to a gentle boil.
6. Now adjust the heat to medium-low and simmer, covered for 15-20 minutes or until done completely.
7. Serve with a garnish of coriander.

# Mushroom Curry

Servings|4   Time|30 minutes
**Nutritional Content (per serving):**
Cal| 160 Fat| 11.9g Protein| 4.9g Carbs| 10.6g Fibre| 2.5g Cholesterol| 0mg

## Ingredients:

- ❖ Olive oil (30 millilitres)
- ❖ Salt and ground black pepper, as required
- ❖ Unsweetened coconut milk (125 millilitres)
- ❖ Fresh parsley (10 grams, chopped)
- ❖ Onions (2, chopped)
- ❖ Garlic cloves (3, minced)
- ❖ Fresh mushrooms (455 grams, chopped)
- ❖ Low-sodium vegetable broth (60 millilitres)

## Directions:

1. In a large-sized wok, heat oil over medium heat and sauté the onion and garlic for 4-5 minutes.
2. Add the mushrooms, salt, and black pepper and cook for 4-5 minutes.
3. Add the broth and coconut milk and bring to a gentle boil.
4. Simmer for 4-5 minutes or until desired doneness.
5. Stir in the coriander and remove from heat.
6. Serve hot.

# Tempeh with Peppers

Servings|2   Time|26 minutes
**Nutritional Content (per serving):**
Cal| 358 Fat| 19.8g Protein| 23.7g Carbs| 28.8g Fibre| 3.3g Cholesterol| 0mg

## Ingredients:

- Balsamic vinegar (15 millilitres)
- Sugar-free tomato sauce (30 grams)
- Garlic powder (2½ grams)
- Olive oil (15 millilitres)
- Small Peppers (2, seeded and chopped)
- Low-sodium soy sauce (15 millilitres)
- Light maple syrup (5 grams)
- Red pepper flakes (1½ grams)
- Tempeh (225 grams, cubed)
- Medium onion (1, chopped)

## Directions:

1. In a small bowl, add the vinegar, soy sauce, tomato sauce, maple syrup, garlic powder and red pepper flakes and beat until well blended. Set aside.
2. In a large-sized wok, heat 15 millilitres of oil over medium heat and cook the tempeh about 2-3 minutes per side.
3. Add the onion and peppers and heat for about 2-3 minutes.
4. Stir in the sauce mixture and cook for about 3-5 minutes, stirring frequently.
5. Serve hot.

# Tofu with Brussels Sprout

Servings|2   Time|30 minutes
**Nutritional Content (per serving):**
Cal| 280 Fat| 19.3g Protein| 14.4g Carbs| 19g Fibre| 5.5g Cholesterol| 0mg

## Ingredients:

- Olive oil (15 millilitres, divided)
- Garlic clove (1, chopped)
- Garlic clove (1, chopped)
- Walnuts (25 grams, chopped)
- Brussels sprouts (225 grams, trimmed and quartered)
- Extra-firm tofu (150 grams, drained, pressed and cut into slices)
- Light maple syrup (20 grams)
- Fresh coriander (5 grams, chopped)

## Directions:

1. In a wok, heat half of the oil over medium heat and sauté the tofu for about 6-7 minutes or until golden brown.
2. Add the garlic and walnuts and sauté for about 1 minute.
3. Add the maple syrup and cook for about 2 minutes.
4. Stir in the coriander and remove from heat.
5. Transfer tofu onto a plate and set aside
6. In the same wok, heat remaining oil over medium-high heat and cook the Brussels sprouts and peppers for about 5 minutes.
7. Stir in the tofu and remove from heat.
8. Serve immediately.

# Quinoa with Asparagus

Servings|2   Time|25 minutes
**Nutritional Content (per serving):**
Cal| 238 Fat| 10g Protein| 10.3g Carbs| 38.8g Fibre| 6.2g Cholesterol| 13mg

## Ingredients:

- Fresh asparagus (225 grams, trimmed)
- Garlic clove (1, minced)
- Ground turmeric (10 grams)
- Low-fat Parmesan cheese (30 grams, grated)
- Olive oil (10 millilitres)
- Small onion (½, chopped)
- Cooked quinoa (95 grams)
- Low-sodium vegetable broth (60 millilitres)
- Fresh lime juice (5 millilitres)

## Directions:

1. In a large-sized saucepan of boiling water, cook the asparagus for about 2-3 minutes.
2. Drain the asparagus well and rinse under cold water.
3. Meanwhile, in a large-sized wok, heat the oil over medium heat and sauté the onion and garlic for about 5 minutes.
4. Stir in the quinoa, turmeric and broth and cook for about 5-6 minutes.
5. Stir in the cheese, lime juice and asparagus and cook for about 3-4 minutes.
6. Serve hot.

# Pasta with Asparagus

Servings|2   Time|22 minutes
**Nutritional Content (per serving):**
Cal| 381 Fat| 18.8g Protein| 12.4g Carbs| 44.7g Fibre| 6.6g Cholesterol| 15mg

## Ingredients:

- Olive oil (30 millilitres)
- Red pepper flakes (1¼ grams)
- Salt and ground black pepper, as required
- Whole-wheat pasta (115 grams, drained)
- Garlic cloves (2, minced)
- Asparagus (225 grams, trimmed and cut into 1½-inch pieces)
- Low-fat Parmesan cheese (15 grams, shredded)

## Directions:

1. In a large-sized cast-iron wok, heat the oil over medium heat and cook the garlic and red pepper flakes for about 1 minute.
2. Add the asparagus, salt and black pepper and cook for about 8-10 minutes, stirring occasionally.
3. Meanwhile, in a large-sized saucepan of lightly salted boiling water, cook the pasta for about 8-10 minutes or according to package's instructions.
4. Drain the pasta and set aside.
5. In the wok of asparagus, place the hot pasta and cheese and toss to coat well.
6. Serve immediately.

# Dinner Recipes

# Quinoa & Chickpeas Salad

Servings|6   Time|40 minutes
**Nutritional Content (per serving):**
Cal| 222 Fat| 5g Protein| 8.4g Carbs| 37.4g Fibre| 5.4g Cholesterol| 0mg

## Ingredients:

- Low-sodium vegetable broth 420 millilitres
- Salt, as required
- Peppers (2, seeded and chopped)
- Fresh coriander (10 grams, chopped)
- Uncooked quinoa (190 grams, rinsed)
- Cooked chickpeas (250 grams)
- Cucumbers (2, chopped
- Green onion (50 grams, chopped)
- Olive oil (15 millilitres)

## Directions:

1. In a saucepan, add the broth over high heat and bring to a boil.
2. Add the quinoa and salt and cook until boiling.
3. Now adjust the heat to low and simmer, covered for about 15-20 minutes or until all the liquid is absorbed.
4. Remove the saucepan of quinoa from heat and set aside, covered for about 5-10 minutes.
5. Uncover and with a fork, fluff the quinoa.
6. In a large serving bowl, place the quinoa with the remaining ingredients and gently toss to coat.
7. Serve immediately.

# Mixed Beans Salad

Servings|8  Time|15 minutes
**Nutritional Content (per serving):**
Cal|165 Fat| 4.2g Protein| 8.4g Carbs| 25.3g Fibre| 8.1g Cholesterol| 0mg

## Ingredients:

### For Salad:

- Cooked cannellini beans (270 grams)
- Cooked red kidney beans (270 grams)
- Cucumber (300 grams, chopped)
- Red onion (120 grams, chopped)
- Tomato (300 grams, chopped)

### For Dressing:

- Garlic clove (1, minced)
- Shallot (15 grams, minced)
- Lemon zest (5 grams, grated finely)
- Fresh lemon juice (60 millilitres)
- Olive oil (30 millilitres)
- Salt and ground black pepper, as required

## Directions:

1. For salad: in a large-sized salad bowl, add the couscous and remaining ingredients and stir to combine.
2. For dressing: in another small-sized bowl, add all ingredients and beat until well blended.
3. Pour the dressing over the salad and gently toss to coat well.
4. Serve immediately.

# Chicken & Fruit Salad

Servings|4   Time|15 minutes
**Nutritional Content (per serving):**
Cal| 310 Fat| 13.2g Protein| 25.9g Carbs| 23.9g Fibre| 5.2g Cholesterol| 63mg

## Ingredients:

- ❖ Apple cider vinegar (30 millilitres)
- ❖ Salt and ground black pepper, as required
- ❖ Lettuce (300 grams, torn)
- ❖ Fresh strawberries (250 grams, hulled and sliced)
- ❖ Extra-virgin olive oil (30 millilitres)
- ❖ Cooked chicken (325 grams, cubed)
- ❖ Apples (2, cored and chopped)
- ❖ Almonds (25 grams, chopped)

## Directions:

1. For vinaigrette: in a small bowl, add vinegar, oil, salt and black pepper and beat well.
2. For salad: in a large salad bowl, blend together all ingredients.
3. Place vinaigrette over chicken mixture and toss to coat well.
4. Serve immediately.

# Beef & Peach Salad

Servings|6   Time|35 minutes
**Nutritional Content (per serving):**
Cal| 222 Fat| 10.6g Protein| 22.8g Carbs| 9g Fibre| 1.9g Cholesterol| 42mg

## Ingredients:

- ❖ Fresh lemon juice (25 millilitres, divided)
- ❖ Salt and ground black pepper, as required
- ❖ Honey (5 grams)
- ❖ Peaches (3, cored and sliced thinly)
- ❖ Extra-virgin olive oil (25 millilitres, divided)
- ❖ Flank steak (455 grams, trimmed)
- ❖ Fresh baby spinach (200 grams)

## Directions:

1. In a large-sized bowl, blend together 5 millilitres of lemon juice, 10 millilitres of olive oil, salt and black pepper.
2. Add steak and coat with mixture generously.
3. Heat a greased non-stick wok over medium-high heat and cook the steak for 5 minutes per side.
4. Place the steak onto a cutting board for about 9-10 minutes before slicing.
5. Cut the steak into slices diagonally across the grain.
6. In a large-sized bowl, add remaining lemon juice, oil, honey, salt and black pepper and beat well.
7. Add spinach and toss to coat well.
8. Divide spinach mixture onto 4 serving plates.
9. Top with steak and peach slices and serve.

# Salmon & Cucumber Salad

Servings|2   Time|15 minutes
**Nutritional Content (per serving):**
Cal| 282 Fat| 19.6g Protein| 17.6g Carbs| 13.1g Fibre| 2.7g Cholesterol| 33mg

## Ingredients:

- ❖ Cooked salmon (150 grams, chopped)
- ❖ Grape tomatoes (70 grams, quartered)
- ❖ Lettuce (75 grams, torn)
- ❖ Fresh spinach (30 grams, torn)
- ❖ Olive oil (30 millilitres)
- ❖ Cucumber (150 grams, sliced)
- ❖ Pepper (150 grams, seeded and sliced)
- ❖ Green onion (10 grams, chopped)
- ❖ Fresh lemon juice (30 millilitres)

## Directions:

1. In a large-sized salad bowl, place all ingredients and gently toss to coat well.
2. Serve immediately.

# Mixed Veggie Soup

Servings|8 · Time|1 hour
**Nutritional Content (per serving):**
Cal| 108 Fat| 4g Protein| 5.7g Carbs| 14.3g Fibre| 4.6g Cholesterol| 0mg

**Ingredients:**

- Olive oil (30 millilitres)
- Medium onion (1, chopped)
- Celery stalks (2, chopped)
- Small cauliflower florets (455 grams)
- Low-sodium vegetable broth (1920 millilitres)
- Salt, as required
- Medium carrots (4, peeled and chopped)
- Tomatoes (400 grams, finely chopped)
- Small cauliflower florets (455 grams)
- Fresh lemon juice (45 millilitres)

**Directions:**

1. In a large-sized soup pan, heat the oil over medium heat and sauté the carrots, celery and onion for 6 minutes.
2. Add in garlic and sauté for about 1 minute.
3. Add the tomatoes and cook for about 2-3 minutes, crushing with the back of a spoon.
4. Add the vegetables and broth and bring to a boil over high heat.
5. Now adjust the heat to low and cook, covered for about 30-35 minutes.
6. Add in lemon juice and salt and serve hot.

# Beans & Barley Soup

Servings|4   Time|55 minutes
**Nutritional Content (per serving):**
Cal| 294 Fat| 4g Protein| 12.3g Carbs| 54.5g Fibre| 12.4g Cholesterol| 0mg

## Ingredients:

- ❖ Olive oil (15 millilitres)
- ❖ Celery stalks (2, chopped)
- ❖ Fresh rosemary (5 grams, chopped)
- ❖ Tomatoes (600 grams, chopped)
- ❖ Cooked white beans (360 grams)
- ❖ Fresh parsley (5 grams, chopped)
- ❖ Onion (1, chopped)
- ❖ Large carrot (1, peeled and chopped)
- ❖ Garlic cloves (2, minced)
- ❖ Low-sodium vegetable broth (960 millilitres)
- ❖ Pearl barley (200 grams)
- ❖ Fresh lemon juice (30 millilitres)

## Directions:

1. In a large-sized soup pan, heat the oil over medium heat and sauté the onion, celery and carrot for about 4-5 minutes.
2. Add the garlic and rosemary and sauté for about 1 minute.
3. Add the tomatoes and cook for 3-4 minutes, crushing with the back of a spoon.
4. Add the barley and broth and bring to a boil.
5. Now adjust the heat to low and simmer, covered for about 20-25 minutes.
6. Stir in the beans and lemon juice and simmer for about 5 minutes more.
7. Garnish with parsley and serve hot

# Chicken & Tofu Soup

Servings|2   Time|35 minutes
**Nutritional Content (per serving):**
Cal| 162 Fat| 10.7g Protein| 19.4g Carbs| 3.5g Fibre| 1.1g Cholesterol| 35mg

**Ingredients:**

- ❖ Olive oil (5 millilitres)
- ❖ Firm tofu (150 grams, pressed, drained and cubed)
- ❖ Salt and ground white pepper, as required
- ❖ Lean ground chicken (115 grams)
- ❖ Low-sodium chicken broth (480 millilitres)
- ❖ Green onions (2, chopped)

**Directions:**

1. In a large-sized wok, heat olive oil over medium-high heat and cook chicken for about 8-10 minutes.
2. Transfer the chicken into a bowl.
3. In the same wok, add tofu and cook for about 5 minutes or until browned from all sides.
4. In a medium-sized soup pan, add broth over medium-low heat and bring to a gentle boil.
5. Now adjust the heat to low.
6. Stir in cooked chicken, tofu and black pepper and simmer for about 4-5 minutes.
7. Stir in green onions and serve hot.

# Steak & Chickpeas Soup

Servings|4   Time|40 minutes
**Nutritional Content (per serving):**
Cal| 216 Fat| 9.8g Protein| 23.2g Carbs| 8.2g Fibre| 2g Cholesterol| 50mg

## Ingredients:

- Sirloin steak (225 grams, trimmed and cut into bite-sized pieces)
- Large carrot (1, peeled and chopped)
- Medium onion (1, chopped)
- Sugar-free tomato paste (40 grams)
- Low-sodium beef broth (960 millilitres)
- Water (240 millilitres)
- Salt and ground black pepper, as required
- Extra-virgin olive oil (20 grams, divided)
- Large celery stalk (1, sliced)
- Fresh thyme (5 grams, chopped)
- Quick-cooking barley (150 grams)
- f Fresh lemon juice (10 millilitres)

## Directions:

1. Season steak with salt and black pepper.
2. In a Dutch oven, heat 10 millilitres of oil over medium heat and sears teak for about 2-3 minutes.
3. Transfer steak into a bowl.
4. In the same pan, heat remaining oil and sauté carrot, celery and onion for about 4-5 minutes.
5. Add tomato paste and thyme and cook for about 1-2 minutes.
6. Add barley, broth, water and remaining black pepper and bring to a boil.
7. Reduce heat to low and simmer for about 15 minutes.
8. Stir in cooked beef and simmer for about 5 minutes.
9. Stir in lemon juice and serve hot.

# Salmon & Cabbage Soup

Servings|4   Time|40 minutes
**Nutritional Content (per serving):**
Cal| 229Fat| 11.1g Protein| 17g Carbs| 17.9g Fibre| 5.7g Cholesterol| 25mg

**Ingredients:**

- ❖ Olive oil (30 millilitres)
- ❖ Garlic cloves (2, minced)
- ❖ Cabbage head (1, chopped)
- ❖ Low-sodium vegetable broth (1200 millilitres)
- ❖ Fresh coriander (10 grams, minced)
- ❖ Fresh lime juice (30 millilitres)
- ❖ Green onions (2, chopped)

- ❖ Shallot (1, chopped)
- ❖ Jalapeño pepper (1, chopped)
- ❖ Small Peppers (2, seeded and finely chopped)
- ❖ Boneless salmon fillets (2 (115-gram), cubed)
- ❖ Salt and ground black pepper, as required

**Directions:**

1. In a large-sized soup pan, heat oil over medium heat and sauté shallot and garlic for 2-3 minutes.
2. Add cabbage and peppers and sauté for about 3-4 minutes.
3. Add broth and bring to a boil over high heat.
4. Now adjust the heat to medium-low and simmer for about 10 minutes.
5. Add salmon and cook for about 5-6 minutes.
6. Stir in the coriander, lemon juice, salt and black pepper and cook for about 1-2 minutes.
7. Serve hot with the topping of green onion.

# Tofu & Pepper Stew

Servings|6   Time|30 minutes
**Nutritional Content (per serving):**
Cal| 107 Fat| 4.8g Protein| 10.3g Carbs| 8.8g Fibre| 2.3g Cholesterol| 0mg

## Ingredients:

- Garlic (10 grams, peeled)
- Roasted red peppers (1 (150-gram) jar, rinsed, drained and chopped)
- Water (480 millilitres)
- Extra-firm tofu (1 (455-gram) package, pressed, drained and cubed)
- Jalapeño pepper (1, seeded and chopped)
- Low-sodium vegetable broth (480 millilitres)
- Medium Peppers (2, seeded and sliced thinly)
- Frozen baby spinach (1 (280-gram) package, thawed)

## Directions:

1. Add the garlic, jalapeño pepper and roasted red peppers in a clean food processor and pulse until smooth.
2. In a large-sized saucepan, add the puree, broth and water over medium-high heat and cook until boiling.
3. Add the peppers and tofu and stir to combine.
4. Now adjust the heat to medium and cook for about 5 minutes.
5. Stir in the spinach and cook for about 5 minutes.
6. Serve hot.

# Chickpeas Stew

Servings|4   Time|45 minutes
**Nutritional Content (per serving):**
Cal| 183 Fat| 5.1g Protein| 7.3g Carbs| 29.2g Fibre| 6.6g Cholesterol| 0mg

## Ingredients:

- Olive oil (15 millilitres)
- Large carrot (, peeled and chopped)
- Large tomatoes (2, peeled, seeded and finely chopped)
- Cooked chickpeas (330 grams)
- Salt and ground black pepper, as required
- Medium onion (1, chopped)
- Garlic cloves (2, minced)
- Red pepper flakes (5 grams)
- Low-sodium vegetable broth (480 millilitres)
- Fresh spinach (90 grams, chopped)
- Fresh lime juice (15 millilitres)

## Directions:

1. In a large-sized saucepan, heat oil over medium heat and sauté the onion and carrot for about 6 minutes.
2. Stir in the garlic and red pepper flakes and sauté for about 1 minute.
3. Add the tomatoes and cook for about 2-3 minutes.
4. Add the broth and bring to a boil.
5. Now adjust the heat to low and simmer for about 10 minutes.
6. Stir in the chickpeas and simmer for about 5 minutes.
7. Stir in the spinach and simmer for 3-4 minutes more.
8. Stir in the lime juice and seasoning and serve hot.

# Chicken & Spinach Stew

Servings|8   Time|45 minutes
**Nutritional Content (per serving):**
Cal| 300 Fat| 17.4g Protein| 7.3g Carbs| 1.8g Fibre| 1.8g Cholesterol| 77mg

## Ingredients:

- Olive oil (30 millilitres)
- Garlic (10 grams, minced)
- Ground turmeric (5 grams)
- Boneless, skinless chicken thighs (6 (115-gram), cut into 1-inch pieces)
- Salt and ground black pepper, as required
- Fresh spinach (90 grams, chopped)

- Onion (1, chopped)
- Fresh ginger (5 grams, minced)
- Ground cumin (5 grams)
- Paprika (5 grams)
- Tomatoes (4, chopped)
- Unsweetened coconut milk (1 (400-millilitre) can)
- Salt and ground black pepper, as required

## Directions:

1. Heat oil in a large-sized heavy-bottomed pan over medium heat and sauté the onion for about 3-4 minutes.
2. Add the ginger, garlic, and spices, and sauté for about 1 minute.
3. Add the chicken and cook for about 4-5 minutes.
4. Add the tomatoes, coconut milk, salt, and black pepper, and bring to a gentle simmer.
5. Now, adjust the heat to low and simmer, covered for about 10-15 minutes.
6. Stir in the spinach and cook for about 4-5 minutes.
7. Remove from heat and serve hot.

# Ground Turkey Chilli

Servings|6 · Time|1 hour
**Nutritional Content (per serving):**
Cal| 303 Fat| 11.5g Protein| 23.1g Carbs| 30.6g Fibre| 7.9g Cholesterol| 54mg

## Ingredients:

- Olive oil (30 millilitres)
- Onion (1, chopped)
- Garlic cloves (2, chopped)
- Water (480 millilitres)
- Tomatoes (500 grams, finely chopped)
- Cooked red kidney beans (360 grams)
- Green onion (25 grams, chopped)
- Pepper (1, seeded and chopped)
- Lean ground turkey (455 grams)
- Ground cumin (5 grams)
- Ground cinnamon (2½ grams)
- Frozen corn (190 grams, thawed)

## Directions:

1. In a large-sized Dutch oven, heat the olive oil over medium-low heat and sauté pepper, onion and garlic for about 5 minutes.
2. Add turkey and cook for about 5-6 minutes, breaking up the chunks with a wooden spoon.
3. Add water, tomatoes and spices and bring to a boil over high heat.
4. Adjust the heat to medium-low and stir in beans and corn.
5. Simmer, covered for about 30 minutes, stirring occasionally.
6. Serve hot with the topping of green onion.

# Beans & Veggie Chili

Servings|5   Time|2 hours 25 minutes
**Nutritional Content (per serving):**
Cal| 284 Fat| 7.5g Protein| 14.8g Carbs| 42.9g Fibre| 14.9g Cholesterol| 0mg

## Ingredients:

- ❖ Olive oil (30 millilitres)
- ❖ Large Pepper (1, seeded and sliced)
- ❖ Ground cumin (5 grams)
- ❖ Tomatoes (400 grams, finely chopped)
- ❖ Low-sodium vegetable broth (480 millilitres)

- ❖ Onion (1, chopped)
- ❖ Garlic cloves (4, minced)
- ❖ Jalapeño peppers (2, sliced)
- ❖ Red chilli powder (10 grams)
- ❖ Cooked black beans (680 grams)
- ❖ Salt and ground black pepper, as required

## Directions:

1. In a large-sized saucepan, heat the oil over medium-high heat and sauté the onion and peppers for 3-4 minutes.
2. Add the garlic, jalapeño peppers, and spices and sauté for about 1 minute.
3. Add the sweet potato and cook for 4-5 minutes.
4. Add the remaining ingredients and bring to a boil.
5. Now adjust the heat to medium-low and simmer, covered for about 1½-2 hours.
6. Stir in salt and black pepper and serve hot.

# Lentil Chili

Servings|8   Time|2 hours 55 minutes
**Nutritional Content (per serving):**
Cal| 277 Fat| 3.3g Protein| 18.4g Carbs| 44.8g Fibre| 20.5g Cholesterol| 0mg

## Ingredients:

- Olive oil (15 millilitres)
- Medium carrots (3, peeled and chopped)
- Jalapeño pepper (1, seeded and chopped)
- Cayenne pepper (5 grams)
- Salt and ground black pepper, as required
- Low-sodium vegetable broth (1920 millilitres)
- Large onion (1, chopped)
- Celery stalks (4, chopped)
- Garlic cloves (2, minced)
- Dried thyme (10 grams)
- Red chilli powder (15 grams)
- Ground cumin (10 grams)
- Sugar-free tomato paste (75 grams)
- Green onion (50 grams, chopped)

## Directions:

1. In a large-sized saucepan, heat the oil over medium heat and sauté the onion, carrot, and celery for 5 minutes.
2. Add the garlic, jalapeño pepper, thyme, and spices and sauté for about 1 minute.
3. Add the tomato paste, lentils, and broth and bring to a boil.
4. Now adjust the heat to low and simmer for 2-2½ hours.
5. Serve hot with a garnish of green onion.

# Lentils with Kale

Servings|6   Time|35 minutes
**Nutritional Content (per serving):**
Cal| 274 Fat| 5.5g Protein| 16.4g Carbs| 41.4g Fibre| 17.8g Cholesterol| 0mg

## Ingredients:

- Red lentils (315 grams)
- Olive oil (30 millilitres)
- Onion (60 grams, chopped)
- Garlic cloves (2, minced)
- Fresh kale (330 grams, tough ribs removed and chopped)
- Low-sodium vegetable broth (360 millilitres)
- Fresh ginger (5 grams, minced)
- Tomatoes (300 grams, chopped
- Salt and ground black pepper, as required

## Directions:

1. In a saucepan, add the broth and lentils over medium-high heat and bring to a boil.
2. Now adjust the heat to and simmer, covered for about 20 minutes or until almost all the liquid is absorbed.
3. Remove from heat and set aside covered.
4. Meanwhile, in a large-sized wok, heat oil over medium heat and sauté the onion for about 5-6 minutes.
5. Add the ginger and garlic and sauté for about 1 minute.
6. Add tomatoes and kale and cook for about 4-5 minutes.
7. Stir in the lentils, salt and black pepper and remove from heat.
8. Serve hot.

# Barley Pilaf

Servings|4   Time|1 hour 20 minutes
**Nutritional Content (per serving):**
Cal| 194 Fat| 9.1g Protein| 4g Carbs| 26.4g Fibre| 5.5g Cholesterol| 0mg

## Ingredients:

- Pearl barley (100 grams)
- Olive oil (30 millilitres), divided
- Garlic cloves (2, minced)
- Green olives (90 grams, sliced)
- Fresh coriander (10 grams, chopped)
- Low-sodium vegetable broth (240 millilitres)
- Onion (60 grams, chopped)
- Pepper (150 grams, seeded and chopped)

## Directions:

1. In a large-sized saucepan, add the barley and broth over medium-high heat and cook until boiling.
2. Immediately adjust the heat to low and simmer, covered for about 45 minutes or until all the liquid is absorbed.
3. In a large-sized wok, heat 15 millilitres of the oil over medium-high heat and sauté the garlic for about 30 seconds.
4. Stir in the cooked barley and cook for about 3 minutes.
5. Remove the wok of barley from heat and set aside.
6. In another wok, heat the remaining oil over medium heat and sauté the onion for about 7 minutes.
7. Add the olives and pepper and stir fry for about 3 minutes.
8. Stir in remaining ingredients and cook for about 3 minutes.
9. Stir in the barley mixture and cook for about 3 minutes.
10. Serve hot.

# Kidney Beans Curry

Servings|6   Time|40 minutes
**Nutritional Content (per serving):**
Cal| 340 Fat| 15.7g Protein| 13.5g Carbs| 40.4g Fibre| 12.5g Cholesterol| 0mg

## Ingredients:

- Olive oil (60 millilitres)
- Garlic cloves (2, minced)
- Fresh ginger (10 grams, minced)
- Ground turmeric (2½ grams)
- Salt and ground black pepper, as required
- Cooked red kidney beans (540 grams)
- Water (480 millilitres)
- Medium onion (1, finely chopped)
- Ground coriander (5 grams)
- Ground cumin (5 grams)
- Cayenne pepper (1¼ grams)
- Large tomatoes (2, finely chopped)
- Fresh coriander (10 grams, chopped)

## Directions:

1. In a large-sized saucepan, heat the oil over medium heat and sauté the onion, garlic, and ginger for 6-8 minutes.
2. Stir in the spices and cook for about 1-2 minutes.
3. Stir in the tomatoes, kidney beans, and water and bring to a boil over high heat.
4. Now adjust the heat to medium and simmer for 10-15 minutes or until desired thickness.
5. Serve hot with a garnishing of parsley.

# Stuffed Chicken Breast

Servings|4   Time|40 minutes
**Nutritional Content (per serving):**
Cal| 235 Fat| 11.5g Protein| 28.9g Carbs| 4.7g Fibre| 1g Cholesterol| 67mg

## Ingredients:

- Olive oil (15 millilitres)
- Pepperoni pepper (1, seeded and sliced thinly)
- Garlic (5 grams, minced)
- Dried oregano (1½ grams)
- Skinless, boneless chicken breasts (4 (140-gram), butterflied and pounded)
- Small onion (1, chopped)
- Pepper (½, seeded and sliced thinly)
- Fresh spinach (30 grams, chopped)
- Salt and ground black pepper, as required

## Directions:

1. Preheat your oven to 180 °C.
2. Line a baking sheet with parchment paper.
3. In a saucepan, heat the olive oil over medium heat and sauté onion and both peppers for about 1 minute.
4. Add the garlic and spinach and cook for about 2-3 minutes or until just wilted.
5. Stir in oregano, salt and black pepper and remove the saucepan from heat.
6. Place the chicken mixture into the middle of each butterflied chicken breast.
7. Fold each chicken breast over filling to make a little pocket and secure with toothpicks.
8. Arrange the chicken breasts onto the prepared baking sheet.
9. Bake for approximately 18-20 minutes.
10. Serve hot.

# Chicken with Mushrooms

Servings|4 Time|35 minutes
**Nutritional Content (per serving):**
Cal| 235 Fat| 11.5g Protein| 28.9g Carbs| 4.7g Fibre| 1g Cholesterol| 67mg

## Ingredients:

- Skinless, boneless chicken breasts (4 (115-gram))
- Olive oil (30 millilitres)
- Fresh mushrooms (320 grams, sliced)
- Balsamic vinegar (60 millilitres)
- Dried thyme (1¼ grams)
- Salt and ground black pepper, as required
- Garlic cloves (6, chopped)
- Low-sodium chicken broth (180 millilitres)
- Bay leaf (1)

## Directions:

1. Sprinkle the chicken breasts with salt and black pepper.
2. In a large-sized sauté pan, heat the oil over medium-high heat and stir fry chicken for about 3 minutes.
3. Add garlic and flip the chicken breasts.
4. Spread mushrooms over chicken and cook for about 3 minutes, shaking the sauté pan frequently.
5. Add broth, vinegar, bay leaf and thyme and stir to combine.
6. Now adjust the heat to medium-low and simmer, covered for about 10 minutes, flipping chicken occasionally.
7. With a slotted spoon, transfer the chicken onto a warm serving platter and with a piece of foil, cover to keep warm.
8. Place the pan of sauce over medium-high heat and cook, uncovered for about 7 minutes.
9. Remove the pan of mushroom sauce from heat and discard the bay leaf.
10. Place mushroom sauce over chicken and serve hot.

# Steak with Green Beans

Servings|2   Time|35 minutes
**Nutritional Content (per serving):**
Cal| 333 Fat| 16.8g Protein| 37.1g Carbs| 8.6g Fibre| 3.9g Cholesterol| 90mg

## Ingredients:

### For Steak:

- ❖ Sirloin steaks (2 (115-gram), trimmed)
- ❖ Salt and ground black pepper, as required
- ❖ Olive oil (15 millilitres)
- ❖ Garlic clove (1, minced)

### For Green Beans:

- ❖ Fresh green beans (225 grams, trimmed)
- ❖ Extra-virgin olive oil (5 millilitres)
- ❖ Fresh lemon juice (5 millilitres)

## Directions:

1. For steak: sprinkle the steaks with salt and black pepper evenly.
2. In a cast-iron sauté pan, heat the olive oil over high heat and sauté garlic for about 15-20 seconds.
3. Add the steaks and cook for about 3 minutes per side.
4. Flip the steaks and cook for about 3-4 minutes or until desired doneness, flipping once.
5. Meanwhile, for green beans: in a pan of boiling water, arrange a steamer basket.
6. Place the green beans in the steamer basket and steam covered for about 4-5 minutes.
7. Carefully transfer the beans into a bowl.
8. Add olive oil and lemon juice and toss to coat well.
9. Divide green beans onto serving plates.
10. Top each with 1 steak and serve.

# Ground Beef with Mushrooms

Servings|4   Time|40 minutes
**Nutritional Content (per serving):**
Cal| 246 Fat| 15.4g Protein| 24.4g Carbs| 3.7g Fibre| 0.9g Cholesterol| 71mg

## Ingredients:

- Lean ground beef (455 grams)
- Garlic cloves (2, minced)
- Fresh mushrooms (200 grams, sliced)
- Low-sodium beef broth (60 millilitres)
- Olive oil (30 millilitres)
- Onion (½, chopped)
- Fresh basil (5 grams, chopped)
- Balsamic vinegar (30 millilitres)
- Fresh parsley (10 grams, chopped)

## Directions:

1. Heat a large-sized non-stick wok over medium-high heat and cook the Lean ground beef for about 8-10 minutes, breaking up the chunks with a wooden spoon.
2. With a slotted spoon, transfer the beef into a bowl.
3. In the same wok, add the onion and garlic and cook for about 3 minutes.
4. Add the mushrooms and cook for about 5-7 minutes.
5. Add the cooked beef, basil, broth and vinegar and bring to a boil.
6. Adjust the heat to medium-low and simmer for about 3 minutes.
7. Stir in parsley and serve immediately.

# Pork with Peppers

Servings|4   Time|28 minutes
**Nutritional Content (per serving):**
Cal| 361 Fat| 22.1g Protein| 31.2g Carbs| 10.4g Fibre| 2.1g Cholesterol| 83mg

**Ingredients:**

- Fresh ginger (10 grams, finely chopped)
- Olive oil (75 millilitres, divided)
- Pork tenderloin (455 grams, trimmed and sliced thinly)
- Fresh lime juice (15 millilitres)
- Garlic cloves (4, finely chopped)
- Fresh coriander (20 grams, chopped and divided)
- Onions (2, sliced thinly)
- Pepper (1, seeded and sliced thinly)

**Directions:**

1. In a large-sized bowl, blend together ginger, garlic, 10 grams of coriander and 60 millilitres of oil.
2. Add pork and coat with mixture generously.
3. Refrigerate to marinate for about 2 hours.
4. Heat a large-sized wok over medium-high heat and stir fry the pork with marinade for about 4-5 minutes.
5. Transfer the pork into a bowl.
6. In the same wok, heat remaining oil over medium heat and sauté onion for about 3 minutes.
7. Stir in pepper and stir fry for about 3 minutes.
8. Stir in pork, lime juice and remaining coriander and cook for about 2 minutes.
9. Serve hot.

# Salmon with Asparagus

Servings|6   Time|35minutes
**Nutritional Content (per serving):**
Cal| 217 Fat| 12g Protein| 24.9g Carbs| 4.7g Fibre| 2.5g Cholesterol| 51mg

## Ingredients:

- ❖ Salmon fillets (6 (115-gram))
- ❖ Fresh parsley (10 grams, minced)
- ❖ Fresh asparagus (680 grams)

- ❖ Olive oil (30 millilitres)
- ❖ Ginger powder (1¼ grams)
- ❖ Salt and ground black pepper, as required

## Directions:

1. Preheat your oven to 200 °C.
2. Grease a large baking dish.
3. In a large-sized bowl, place all ingredients and mix well.
4. Arrange the salmon fillets into the prepared baking dish in a single layer.
5. Bake for approximately 15-20 minutes or until desired doneness of salmon.
6. Meanwhile, in a pan of boiling water, add asparagus and cook for about 4-5 minutes.
7. Drain the asparagus well.
8. Serve salmon fillets alongside the asparagus.

# Snacks Recipes

# Grilled Watermelon

Servings|4   Time|14 minutes
**Nutritional Content (per serving):**
Cal| 11 Fat| 0.1g Protein| 0.2g Carbs| 2.6g Fibre| 0.2g Cholesterol| 0mg

## Ingredients:

- ❖ Watermelon (1, peeled and cut into 1-inch thick wedges)
- ❖ Pinch of cayenne pepper
- ❖ Garlic clove (1, minced finely)
- ❖ Fresh lime juice (30 millilitres)
- ❖ Pinch of salt

## Directions:

1. Preheat your grill to high heat. Grease the grill grate.
2. Place the watermelon wedges onto the grill and cook for about 2 minutes from both sides.
3. Meanwhile, in a small-sized bowl, blend together remaining ingredients.
4. Drizzle the watermelon wedges with lemon mixture and serve.

# Banana Chips

Servings|4   Time|1 hour 10 minutes
**Nutritional Content (per serving):**
Cal| 61 Fat| 0.2g Protein| 0.7g Carbs| 15.5g Fibre| 1.8g Cholesterol| 0mg

## Ingredients:

- ❖ 1 Large bananas (2, peeled and cut into ¼-inch thick slices)
- ❖ Salt, as required

## Directions:

1. Preheat your oven to 120 °C. Line a large-sized baking sheet with baking paper.
2. Place the banana slices onto the prepared baking sheet in a single layer.
3. Bake for approximately 1 hour.

# Spiced Chickpeas

Servings|12   Time|55 minutes
## Nutritional Content (per serving):
Cal| 78 Fat| 1.9g Protein| 2.8g Carbs| 12.8g Fibre| 2.6g Cholesterol| 0mg

## Ingredients:

- Cooked chickpeas (660 grams)
- Dried oregano (1½ grams, crushed)
- Salt, as required
- Garlic cloves (2, minced)
- Paprika (1½ grams)
- Ground cumin (1¼ grams)
- Olive oil (15 millilitres)

## Directions:

1. Preheat your oven to 200 °C.
2. Grease a large baking sheet.
3. Place chickpeas onto the prepared baking sheet in a single layer.
4. Roast for about 30 minutes, stirring the chickpeas after every 10 minutes.
5. Meanwhile, in a small mixing bowl, blend together garlic, thyme and spices.
6. Remove the baking sheet from oven.
7. Place the garlic mixture and oil over the chickpeas and toss to coat well.
8. Roast for about 10-15 minutes more.
9. Now turn the oven off but leave the baking sheet inside for about 10 minutes before serving.

# Roasted Cashews

Servings|12   Time|20 minutes
**Nutritional Content (per serving):**
Cal| 174 Fat| 14g Protein| 4.7g Carbs| 10g Fibre| 1g Cholesterol| 0mg

## Ingredients:

- ❖ Raw cashews (360 grams)
- ❖ Cayenne pepper (1¼ grams)
- ❖ Pinch of salt
- ❖ Ground cumin (2½ grams)
- ❖ Fresh lemon juice (15 millilitres)

## Directions:

1. Preheat your oven to 200 °C.
2. Line a large roasting pan with a piece of foil.
3. In a large-sized bowl, add the cashews and spices and toss to coat well.
4. Transfer the cashews into the prepared roasting pan.
5. Roast for about 8-10 minutes.
6. Drizzle with lemon juice and serve.

# Strawberry Salsa

Servings|4   Time|15 minutes
**Nutritional Content (per serving):**
Cal| 31 Fat| 0.2g Protein| 0.6g Carbs| 7.4g Fibre| 1.6g Cholesterol| 0mg

## Ingredients:

- Fresh lime juice (30 millilitres)
- Pinch of fine salt
- Fresh strawberries (250 grams, hulled and chopped)
- Small onion (½, chopped)
- Light maple syrup (10 grams)
- Jalapeño pepper (, seeded and chopped)
- Fresh coriander (10 grams, chopped)

## Directions:

1. In a large-sized bowl, add all ingredients and stir to combine.
2. Serve immediately.

# Tomato Salsa

Servings|4   Time|15 minutes
**Nutritional Content (per serving):**
Cal| 65 Fat| 3.9g Protein| 1.5g Carbs| 7.6g Fibre| 2.2g Cholesterol| 0mg

## Ingredients:

- Large tomatoes (3, chopped)
- Fresh coriander (10 grams, chopped)
- Garlic clove (1, minced finely)
- Salt and ground black pepper, as required
- Small onion (1, chopped)
- Jalapeño pepper (1, seeded and minced)
- Fresh lime juice (30 millilitres)
- Olive oil (15 millilitres)

## Directions:

1. In a large-sized bowl, add all the ingredients and gently toss to coat well.
2. Serve immediately.

# Strawberry Gazpacho

Servings|4   Time|15 minutes
**Nutritional Content (per serving):**
Cal| 111 Fat| 4.2g Protein| 2.1g Carbs| 18.7g Fibre| 4.3g Cholesterol| 0mg

## Ingredients:

- Fresh strawberries (680 grams, hulled and sliced)
- Small cucumber (1, peeled, seeded and chopped)
- Small garlic clove (1, chopped)
- Olive oil (15 millilitres)
- Balsamic vinegar (45 millilitres)
- Red Pepper (75 grams, seeded and chopped)
- Onion (30 grams, chopped)
- Fresh basil leaves (10 grams)
- Jalapeño pepper (¼, seeded and chopped)

## Directions:

1. In a high-power blender, add all the ingredients and pulse until smooth.
2. Transfer the gazpacho into a large-sized bowl.
3. Cover and refrigerate to chill completely before serving.

# Avocado Gazpacho

Servings|6   Time|15 minutes
**Nutritional Content (per serving):**
Cal| 218 Fat| 19.9g Protein| 3.2g Carbs| 9.8g Fibre| 7g Cholesterol| 0mg

## Ingredients:

- Large avocados (3, peeled, pitted and chopped)
- Low-sodium vegetable broth (720 millilitres)
- Ground cumin (5 grams)
- Fresh coriander (15 grams)
- Fresh lemon juice (30 millilitres)
- Cayenne pepper (1¼ grams)
- Salt, as required

## Directions:

1. Add all ingredients in a high-power blender and pulse until smooth.
2. Transfer the soup into a large-sized bowl.
3. Cover the bowl and refrigerate to chill for at least 2-3 hours before serving.

# Chickpeas Hummus

Servings|12   Time|10 minutes
**Nutritional Content (per serving):**
Cal| 171 Fat| 10.4g Protein| 5.5g Carbs| 15.9g Fibre| 3.9g Cholesterol| 0mg

## Ingredients:

- ❖ Cooked chickpeas (660 grams)
- ❖ Garlic clove (1, chopped)
- ❖ Salt, as required
- ❖ Water, as required

- ❖ Pinch of cayenne pepper
- ❖ Tahini (190 grams)
- ❖ Fresh lemon juice (30 millilitres
- ❖ Olive oil (15 millilitres)

## Directions:

1. In a high-power blender, add all ingredients except for oil and cayenne pepper and pulse until smooth.
2. Transfer the hummus into a large-sized bowl and drizzle with oil.
3. Sprinkle with cayenne pepper and serve immediately.

# Cauliflower Hummus

Servings|6   Time|20 minutes
**Nutritional Content (per serving):**
Cal| 58 Fat| 5.3g Protein| 1.1g Carbs| 2.9g Fibre| 1.2g Cholesterol| 0mg

## Ingredients:

- Medium cauliflower head (1, trimmed and chopped)
- Olive oil (30 millilitres)
- Fresh chives (5 grams, minced)
- Garlic cloves (2, chopped)
- Almond butter (30 grams)
- Salt, as required
- Pinch of cayenne pepper

## Directions:

1. In a large-sized saucepan of boiling water add the cauliflower and cook over medium heat for about 4-5 minutes.
2. Drain the cauliflower well and set aside to cool it slightly.
3. In a clean food processor, add the cauliflower, garlic, almond butter, oil, and salt and pulse until smooth.
4. Transfer the hummus into a serving bowl.
5. Sprinkle with chives and cayenne pepper and serve immediately.

# Cinnamon Cookies

Servings|8   Time|40 minutes

**Nutritional Content (per serving):**

Cal| 258 Fat| 24.9g Protein| 6g Carbs| 6g Fibre| 3.5g Cholesterol| 20mg

## Ingredients:

- ❖ Almond meal (200 grams)
- ❖ Egg (1)
- ❖ Liquid stevia (5 millilitres)
- ❖ Vanilla extract (5 millilitres)
- ❖ Ground cinnamon (5 grams)
- ❖ Coconut oil (95-100 grams, softened)

## Directions:

1. Preheat your oven to 150 °C.
2. Grease a large-sized cookie sheet.
3. In a large-sized bowl, add all ingredients and mix until well blended.
4. Make small equal-sized balls.
5. Arrange the balls onto the prepared cookie sheet about 2-inch apart.
6. Bake for approximately 5 minutes.
7. Remove the cookie sheet from oven and with a fork, press down each ball.
8. Bake or about 18-20 minutes.
9. Remove the cookie sheet from oven and place onto a wire rack to cool for about 5 minutes.
10. Then invert the cookies onto the wire rack to cool completely before serving.

# Pecan Cookies

Servings|6   Time|29 minutes
**Nutritional Content (per serving):**
Cal| 152 Fat| 13.9g Protein| 3.8g Carbs| 5.1g Fibre| 3.1g Cholesterol| 55mg

## Ingredients:

- Eggs (2)
- Coconut oil (10 grams, melted)
- Coconut flour (5 grams)
- Unsweetened coconut (95 grams, shredded)
- Almond butter (120 grams)
- Vanilla extract (2½ millilitres)
- Ground cinnamon (5 grams)
- Pecans (30 grams, finely chopped)

## Directions:

1. Preheat your oven to 180 ºC.
2. Line a large-sized cookie sheet with a large parchment paper.
3. In a large-sized bowl. add the eggs, almond butter and coconut oil and beat until well blended.
4. Add the flour and cinnamon and mix until well blended.
5. Fold in the coconut and pecans.
6. Spoon the mixture onto the prepared cookie sheet in a single layer.
7. With your hands, flatten each cookie slightly.
8. Bake for approximately 12-14 minutes or until top becomes golden brown.
9. Remove the cookie sheet from oven and place onto a wire rack to cool for about 5 minutes.
10. Then invert the cookies onto the wire rack to cool completely before serving.

# Fennel Cookies

Servings|5   Time|24 minutes
**Nutritional Content (per serving):**
Cal| 136 Fat| 10.8g Protein| 1.1g Carbs| 9.3g Fibre| 3.2g Cholesterol| 0mg

## Ingredients:

- Coconut flour (35 grams)
- Pinch of ground cinnamon
- Pinch of ground cloves
- Coconut oil (50 grams, softened)
- Fresh ginger root (5 grams, grated finely)
- Whole fennel seeds (1¼ grams)
- Pinch of ground cardamom
- Pinch of salt and ground black pepper
- Light maple syrup (35 grams)
- Vanilla extract (5 millilitres)

## Directions:

1. Preheat your oven to 185 °C.
2. Line a cookie sheet with parchment paper.
3. In a large-sized bowl, add the flour, fennel seeds, spices, salt and black pepper and mix well.
4. In another bowl, add the coconut oil, maple syrup and vanilla extract and beat until well blended.
5. Add the ginger and stir to combine.
6. Add the flour mixture and mix until a smooth dough forms.
7. Make small equal-sized balls from the mixture.
8. Arrange the balls onto the prepared cookie sheet in a single layer about 1-inch apart and with your fingers, gently press down each ball to form the cookies.
9. Bake for approximately 9 minutes or until golden brown.
10. Remove the cookie sheet from oven and place onto a wire rack to cool for about 5 minutes.
11. Then invert the cookies onto the wire rack to cool completely before serving.

# Seeds Crackers

Servings|15  Time|12¼ hours
**Nutritional Content (per serving):**
Cal| 113 Fat| 8g Protein| 3.9g Carbs| 5.7g Fibre| 4.7g Cholesterol| 0mg

**Ingredients:**

- Water (480 millilitres)
- Flaxseeds (150 grams)
- Light maple syrup (5 grams)
- Fresh lemon juice (60 millilitres)
- Sunflower seeds (140 grams)
- Fresh ginger (10 grams, chopped)
- Ground turmeric (5 grams)
- Pinch of salt

**Directions:**

1. In a bowl, add water, sunflower seeds and flaxseeds and soak overnight.
2. Drain the seeds.
3. In a clean food processor, add soaked seeds and remaining ingredients and pulse until well blended.
4. Set dehydrator at 45 °C.
5. Line a dehydrator tray with unbleached parchment paper.
6. Place the mixture onto the prepared dehydrator tray evenly.
7. With a knife, score the size of crackers.
8. Dehydrate for about 12 hours.

# Celery Crackers

Servings|12   Time|2¼ hours
**Nutritional Content (per serving):**
Cal| 244 Fat| 16.6g Protein| 7.1g Carbs| 11.7g Fibre| 10.8g Cholesterol| 0mg

## Ingredients:

- Celery stalks (10)
- Fresh thyme leaves (5 grams)
- Apple cider vinegar (30 millilitres)
- Olive oil (60 millilitres)
- Fresh rosemary leaves (5 grams)
- Salt, as required
- Flaxseeds (450 grams, roughly ground)

## Directions:

1. Preheat your oven to 110 °C.
2. Line 2 large-sized baking sheets with parchment paper.
3. In a clean food processor, add all ingredients except for flaxseeds and pulse until a puree form.
4. Add flaxseeds and pulse until well blended.
5. Transfer the dough into a bowl and set aside for about 2-3 minutes.
6. Divide the dough in 2 portions.
7. Place 1 portion in each prepared baking sheet evenly.
8. With the back of a spatula, smooth and press the dough to ¼-inch thickness.
9. With a knife, score the squares in the dough.
10. Bake for approximately 1 hour.
11. Flip the side and bake for 1 hour more.
12. Remove the baking sheets of crackers from oven and set aside to cool for about 15 minutes.

# Almond Scones

Servings|6   Time|30 minutes
**Nutritional Content (per serving):**
Cal| 357 Fat| 30.3g Protein| 4.7g Carbs| 13.8g Fibre| 4.7g Cholesterol| 27mg

## Ingredients:

- Almonds (100 grams)
- Arrowroot flour (30 grams)
- Ground turmeric (5 grams)
- Egg (1)
- Olive oil (60 millilitres)
- Vanilla extract (5 millilitres)
- Almond flour (140 grams)
- Coconut flour (5 grams)
- Salt and ground black pepper, as required
- Light maple syrup (55 grams)

## Directions:

1. Preheat your oven to 180 °C.
2. In a clean food processor, add almonds and pulse until chopped roughly
3. Transfer the chopped almonds into a large-sized bowl.
4. Add flours and spices and mix well.
5. In another bowl, add remaining ingredients and beat until well blended.
6. Add flour mixture into egg mixture and mix until well blended.
7. Arrange a plastic wrap over cutting board.
8. Place the dough over the cutting board.
9. With your hands, pat into 2½-centimetre thick circle.
10. Carefully cut the circle into 6 wedges.
11. Arrange the scones onto a cookie sheet in a single layer.
12. Bake for approximately 15-20 minutes.

# Tomato Bruschetta

Servings|6   Time|19 minutes
**Nutritional Content (per serving):**
Cal| 77 Fat| 1.6g Protein| 3.2g Carbs| 13.4g Fibre| 2.3g Cholesterol| 0mg

## Ingredients:

- ❖ Whole-grain baguette (½)
- ❖ Fennel (45 grams, chopped)
- ❖ Fresh parsley (5 grams, chopped)
- ❖ Salt and ground black pepper, as required

- ❖ Tomatoes (3, chopped)
- ❖ Garlic cloves (2, minced)
- ❖ Fresh basil (5 grams, chopped)
- ❖ Balsamic vinegar (10 millilitres)
- ❖ Olive oil (5 millilitres)

## Directions:

1. Preheat your oven to broiler.
2. Arrange a rack in the top portion of the oven.
3. Cut the bread into 6 (½-inch-thick) slices diagonally.
4. Arrange the bread slices onto a baking sheet in a single layer.
5. Broil for about 2 minutes per side.
6. Meanwhile, in a bowl, add remaining ingredients and toss to coat.
7. Place the tomato mixture on each toasted bread slice evenly and serve immediately.

# Chicken Popcorn

Servings|3   Time|40 minutes
**Nutritional Content (per serving):**
Cal| 352 Fat| 24.7g Protein| 25.4g Carbs| 4.6g Fibre| 1.6g Cholesterol| 74mg

## Ingredients:

- ❖ 1 Boneless, skinless chicken thigh (250 grams, cut into bite-sized pieces)
- ❖ Salt and ground black pepper, as required
- ❖ Olive oil (15 millilitres)
- ❖ Unsweetened coconut milk (200 millilitres)
- ❖ Ground turmeric (5 grams)
- ❖ Coconut flour (10 grams)
- ❖ Desiccated coconut (20 grams)

## Directions:

1. In a large-sized bowl, blend together chicken, coconut milk, turmeric, salt and black pepper.
2. Cover and refrigerate to marinate overnight.
3. Preheat your oven to 200 ºC.
4. In a shallow dish, blend together coconut flour and desiccated coconut.
5. Coat the chicken pieces in coconut mixture evenly.
6. Arrange chicken pieces onto a baking sheet and drizzle with oil evenly.
7. Bake for approximately 20-25 minutes.
8. Serve warm.

# Chicken Nuggets

Servings|8   Time|45 minutes
**Nutritional Content (per serving):**
Cal| 166 Fat| 9.5g Protein| 14.1g Carbs| 3.2g Fibre| 1.7g Cholesterol| 74mg

## Ingredients:

- Skinless, boneless chicken breasts (455 grams, cut into 2x1-inch chunks)
- Onion powder (2½ grams)
- Salt and ground black pepper, as required
- Eggs (2)
- Almond flour (100 grams)
- Dried oregano (5 grams)
- Garlic powder (2½ grams)
- Paprika (2½ grams)

## Directions:

1. Preheat your oven to 180 ºC.
2. Grease a baking sheet.
3. In a shallow bowl, whisk the eggs.
4. In another shallow bowl, place the flour, oregano, spices, salt, and black pepper and mix until well blended.
5. Dip the chicken nuggets in beaten eggs and then coat with the flour mixture.
6. Arrange the chicken nuggets onto the prepared baking sheet in a single layer.
7. Bake for approximately 30 minutes or until golden brown.
8. Remove the baking sheet of nuggets from oven and set aside to cool slightly.
9. Serve warm.

# Chicken Fingers

Servings|6   Time|33 minutes
**Nutritional Content (per serving):**
Cal| 177 Fat| 9.4g Protein| 20.5g Carbs| 3.3g Fibre| 1.7g Cholesterol| 71mg

## Ingredients:

- Skinless, boneless chicken breasts (455 grams, cut into strips)
- Paprika (1½ grams)
- Garlic powder (1½ grams)
- Almond meal (70 grams)
- Ground turmeric (2½ grams)
- Cayenne pepper (1½ grams)
- Salt and ground black pepper, as required

## Directions:

1. Preheat your oven to 190 ºC.
2. Line a large-sized baking sheet with parchment paper.
3. In a shallow dish, beat the egg.
4. In another shallow dish, blend together almond meal and spices.
5. Dip each chicken strip into egg and then coat with spice mixture evenly
6. Arrange the chicken strips onto the prepared baking sheet in a single layer.
7. Bake for approximately 16-18 minutes.

# Cod Sticks

Servings|4   Time|27 minutes
**Nutritional Content (per serving):**
Cal| 155 Fat| 8.2g Protein| 15g Carbs| 2.4g Fibre| 1.4g Cholesterol| 83mg

## Ingredients:

- ❖ Large egg (1)
- ❖ Dried parsley (5 grams)
- ❖ Salt and ground black pepper, as required
- ❖ Almond flour (50 grams)
- ❖ Cayenne pepper (1¼ grams)
- ❖ Cod fillets (300 grams, sliced thinly)

## Directions:

1. Preheat your oven to 180 ºC.
2. Lightly grease a large-sized baking sheet.
3. In a shallow dish, whisk the egg.
4. In another shallow dish, blend together flour, parsley, cayenne pepper, salt and black pepper.
5. Dip the fish sticks in egg and then coat with flour mixture completely.
6. Arrange the chicken strips onto the prepared baking sheet in a single layer.
7. Bake for approximately 10-12 minutes, flipping once halfway through.
8. Serve warm.

# Broccoli Tots

Servings|6   Time|50 minutes
**Nutritional Content (per serving):**
Cal| 235 Fat| 17.8g Protein| 9.7g Carbs| 7.6g Fibre| 3.4g Cholesterol| 109mg

## Ingredients:

- Frozen chopped broccoli (1 (355-gram) package)
- Cayenne pepper (2½ grams)
- Low-fat cheddar cheese (115 grams, grated)
- Olive oil cooking spray
- Large eggs (3)
- Dried oregano (1½ grams)
- Salt and ground white pepper, as required
- Almond flour (100 grams)

## Directions:

1. Preheat your oven to 200 °C.
2. Line two baking sheets with lightly greased parchment paper.
3. In a microwave-safe bowl, place the broccoli and microwave, covered for about 5 minutes, stirring once halfway through.
4. Drain the broccoli well.
5. In a large-sized bowl, place the eggs, oregano, garlic powder, cayenne pepper, red pepper flakes, salt and white pepper and beat until well blended.
6. Add the cooked broccoli, cheddar cheese and almond flour and mix until well blended.
7. With slightly wet hands, make 24 equal-sized patties from the mixture.
8. Arrange the patties onto prepared baking sheets in a single layer about 2-inch apart.
9. Lightly spray each patty with the cooking spray.
10. Bake for approximately 15 minutes per side or until golden brown from both sides.
11. Serve warm.

# Veggie Latkes

Servings|4   Time|35 minutes
**Nutritional Content (per serving):**
Cal| 300 Fat| 22g Protein| 4.3g Carbs| 17.2g Fibre| 4.4g Cholesterol| 82mg

## Ingredients:

- Arrowroot powder (30 grams)
- Salt and ground black pepper, as required
- Medium Courgettes (2, shredded)
- Jalapeño pepper (1, finely chopped)
- Almond flour (100 grams)
- Medium carrot (1, peeled and shredded)
- Small onion (1, chopped)
- Small garlic cloves (2, minced)
- Eggs (2, beaten)
- Olive oil (30 millilitres)

## Directions:

1. In a large-sized bowl, blend together arrowroot powder, almond flour, salt and black pepper.
2. Add remaining ingredients except for oil and mix until well blended.
3. Divide mixture into 8 equal-sized portions.
4. In a large-sized non-stick wok, heat oil over medium heat and cook 4 latkes for about 2-3 minutes.
5. Flip the side and cook for about 2 minutes more.
6. Repeat with the remaining latkes.
7. Serve warm.

# Courgette Sticks

Servings|8   Time|80 minutes
**Nutritional Content (per serving):**
Cal| 86 Fat| 6.2g Protein| 5.5g Carbs| 3.5g Fibre| 1.3g Cholesterol| 47mg

**Ingredients:**

- Courgettes (2, cut into 7½-centimetre sticks lengthwise)
- Low-fat Parmesan cheese (55 grams, grated)
- Italian seasoning (2½ grams)
- Salt, as required
- Eggs (2)
- Almonds (50 grams, finely ground)

**Directions:**

1. In a large-sized colander, place courgette sticks and sprinkle with salt. Set aside for about 1 hour to drain.
2. Preheat your oven to 220 °C.
3. Line a large-sized baking sheet with parchment paper.
4. Squeeze the courgette sticks to remove excess liquid.
5. With a paper towel, pat dry the courgette sticks.
6. In a shallow dish, whisk the eggs.
7. In another shallow dish, blend together remaining ingredients.
8. Dip the courgette sticks in egg and then coat with the cheese mixture evenly.
9. Arrange the courgette sticks onto the prepared baking sheet in a single layer.
10. Bake for approximately 25 minutes, turning once halfway through.
11. Serve warm.

# Apple Leather

Servings|4   Time|12 hours 25 minutes
**Nutritional Content (per serving):**
Cal| 286 Fat| 1.1g Protein| 1.6g Carbs| 76.1g Fibre| 14.3g Cholesterol| 0mg

## Ingredients:

- ❖ 1 Water (240 millilitres)
- ❖ Ground cinnamon (10 grams)
- ❖ Fresh lemon juice (30 millilitres)
- ❖ Apples (960 grams, peeled, cored and chopped)

## Directions:

1. In a large-sized pan, add water and apples over medium-low heat and simmer for about 10-15 minutes, stirring occasionally.
2. Remove the pan of apples from heat and let them cool slightly.
3. In a high-power blender, add apple mixture and pulse until smooth.
4. Return the mixture into pan over medium-low heat.
5. Stir in cinnamon and lemon juice and simmer for about 10 minutes.
6. Transfer the mixture onto dehydrator trays and with the back of the spoon smooth the top.
7. Set the dehydrator at 60 °C.
8. Dehydrate for about 10-12 hours.
9. Cut the apple leather into equal-sized rectangles.
10. Now roll each rectangle to make fruit rolls.

# 28 Days Meal Plan

## Day 1:

**Breakfast:** Blueberry Chia Pudding

**Lunch:** Orange & Kale Salad

**Snack:** Grilled Watermelon

**Dinner:** Pork with Peppers

## Day 2:

**Breakfast:** Seeds Porridge

**Lunch:**   Turkey Burgers

**Snack:** Strawberry Salsa

**Dinner:** Kidney Beans Curry

## Day 3:

**Breakfast:** Kiwi smoothie

**Lunch:** Tomato Soup

**Snack:** Pecan Cookies

**Dinner:** Chicken & Fruit Salad

## Day 4:

**Breakfast:** Oatmeal & Yoghurt Bowl

**Lunch:** Cauliflower Soup

**Snack:** Celery Crackers

**Dinner:** Mixed Veggie Soup

## Day 5:

**Breakfast:** Quinoa Bread

**Lunch:** Beef Burgers

**Snack:** Cauliflower Hummus

**Dinner:** Beans & Barley Soup

## Day 6:

**Breakfast:** Blueberry Muffins

**Lunch:** Broccoli Soup

**Snack:** Banana Chips

**Dinner:** Ground Beef with Mushrooms

## Day 7:

**Breakfast:** Banana Sandwich

**Lunch:** Aubergine Curry

**Snack:** Chicken Popcorn

**Dinner:** Stuffed Chicken Breasts

## Day 8:

**Breakfast:** Beet & Berries Smoothie Bowl

**Lunch:** Tofu with Brussels Sprout

**Snack:** Cinnamon Cookies

**Dinner:** Mixed Beans Salad

## Day 9:

**Breakfast:** Quinoa Bread

**Lunch:** Veggie Kebabs

**Snack:** Strawberry Gazpacho

**Dinner:** Chicken & Tofu Soup

## Day 10:

**Breakfast:** Apple Porridge

**Lunch:** Beef Burgers

**Snack:** Spiced Chickpeas

**Dinner:** Barley Pilaf

## Day 11:

**Breakfast:** Spiced Quinoa Porridge

**Lunch:**

**Snack:** Chicken Fingers

**Dinner:** Beef & Peach Salad

## Day 12:

**Breakfast:** Blueberry Oatmeal

**Lunch:** Turkey Burgers

**Snack:** Courgette Sticks

**Dinner:** Chickpeas Stew

## Day 13:

**Breakfast:** Blueberry Waffles

**Lunch:** Quinoa with Asparagus

**Snack:** Tomato Bruschetta

**Dinner:** Pork with Peppers

## Day 14:

**Breakfast:** Berries Muesli

**Lunch:** Vegetarian Taco Bowl

**Snack:** Roasted Cashews

**Dinner:** Ground Turkey chilli

## Day 15:

**Breakfast:** Avocado & Chickpeas Toast

**Lunch:** Tuna Stuffed Avocado

**Snack:** Strawberry Salsa

**Dinner:** Tofu & Pepper Stew

## Day 16:

**Breakfast:** Buckwheat Porridge

**Lunch:** Broccoli with Peppers

**Snack:** Veggie Latkes

**Dinner:** Salmon & Cabbage Soup

## Day 17:

**Breakfast:** Courgette Bread

**Lunch:** Pasta with Asparagus

**Snack:** Cod Sticks

**Dinner:** Lentils with Kale

## Day 18:

**Breakfast:** Kale Muffins

**Lunch:** Cucumber & Tomato Salad

**Snack:** Apple Leather

**Dinner:** Stuffed Chicken Breast

## Day 19:

**Breakfast:** Banana Pancakes

**Lunch:** Chicken Lettuce Wraps

**Snack:** Fennel Cookies

**Dinner:** Quinoa & Chickpeas Salad

## Day 20:

**Breakfast:** Baked Oatmeal

**Lunch:** Asparagus Soup

**Snack:** Chickpeas Hummus

**Dinner:** Steak with Green Beans

## Day 21:

**Breakfast:** Bulgur Porridge

**Lunch:** Mushroom Curry

**Snack:** Almond Scones

**Dinner:** Chicken & Spinach Stew

## Day 22:

**Breakfast:** Strawberry & Banana Smoothie Bowl

**Lunch:** Tempeh with Peppers

**Snack:** Grilled Watermelon

**Dinner:** Salmon & Cucumber Salad

## Day 23:

**Breakfast:** Blueberry Waffles

**Lunch:** Chickpeas Stuffed Avocado

**Snack:** Broccoli Tots

**Dinner:** Beans & Veggie Chili

## Day 24:

**Breakfast:** Tofu & Veggie Scramble

**Lunch:** Nutty Brussels Sprout

**Snack:** Pecan Cookies

**Dinner:** Chicken with Mushrooms

## Day 25:

**Breakfast:** Kale Smoothie

**Lunch:** Salmon Lettuce Wraps

**Snack:** Seed Crackers

**Dinner:** Beans & Barley Soup

## Day 26:

**Breakfast:** Buckwheat Porridge

**Lunch:** Tofu & Oat Burgers

**Snack:** Avocado Gazpacho

**Dinner:** Steak & Chickpeas Soup

## Day 27:

**Breakfast:** Vanilla Pancakes

**Lunch:** Apple & Strawberry Salad

**Snack:** Chicken Nuggets

**Dinner:** Lentil Chili

## Day 28:

**Breakfast:** Quinoa Porridge

**Lunch:** Broccoli Soup

**Snack:** Tomato Salsa

**Dinner:** Salmon with Asparagus

# Index

Printed in Great Britain
by Amazon